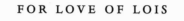
FOR LOVE OF LOIS

For Love of Lois

EDWARD BLISS JR.

Fordham University Press

New York

Library of Congress Cataloging-in-Publication Data

Bliss, Edward, 1912-2002

   For love of Lois / Edward Bliss, Jr.—1st ed.

      p. cm.

   ISBN 0-8232-2265-9 (hard cover)

   1. Bliss, Lois—Mental health. 2. Alzheimer's disease—Patients—Biography. 3. Alzheimer's disease—Patients—Care.

I. Title.

   RC523.2.B556 2003

   362.1'96831'0092—dc21

                        2003002747

Printed in the United States of America

07 06 05 04 03 5 4 3 2 1

First Edition

*To all those who work for a world
without Alzheimer's disease.*

CONTENTS

"If you can keep your head when all about you are losing theirs . . ." That line of Kipling's used to pop into my head so many times during the years I spent with Ed Bliss.

Ed was the top editor at CBS News. Ed Murrow's brilliant copy went through Ed's hands before broadcast, and later I was blessed by inheriting his talents for the CBS Evening News. Many of the hours preparing for a news broadcast are hectic, and frequently the last minutes can be positively chaotic. Those who lost their heads were numerous, I among them. But throughout the newsroom pandemonium, Ed was the seemingly impassive impresario whose unflappable calm seemed to guarantee to all of us that the broadcast would get on the air.

Ed's gentlemanly behavior set him apart and cloaked him with a dignity in an environment of flamboyance that tinged so many of us broadcast journalists. For one thing, I don't believe I ever heard a word of profanity escape his lips—which undoubtedly could be attributed to his childhood as the son of a missionary to remote villages in China.

He and Lois were delightful dinner companions, intelligent observers of the sometimes topsy-turvy world in which we lived as journalists. Ed left the CBS newsroom to become a professor of journalism at American University in Washington, D.C.

He turned out to be, as we all expected, as successful a teacher as he had been an editor. After all, in the latter capacity he had been, in many ways and to many freshmen journalists, nine-tenths teacher. His students apparently adored him and, as successful reporters and broadcasters around the world, they still sing his praises.

This book is something of a surprise. While there was no mistaking his devotion to Lois, and her devotion to him, Ed Bliss hardly seemed the type to bare his soul to public examination. The fact that he wrote this book is testimony to the depth of the emotions that gripped him in the loneliness of Lois's departure.

The title gives it away. This is, indeed, a love story. A lovely love story. There are undoubtedly many couples whose romance lives, grows, and blossoms during their lifetimes. We can hope for our society and our civilization that they are in the majority. But, seldom are we reminded of this happy fact: it's not until a lover like Ed Bliss comes along and spills onto the written page the deep passion with which he and Lois lived their lives together that we can appreciate such a lifelong devotion.

The passion is not that of a cheap novel, but the deep appreciation that only in the presence of each other is life complete. This fundamental of their relationship is brought sharply into focus as the threat of separation begins to shadow their existence.

This is destined to be the final chapter for most of us. Ed Bliss captures each moment of this emotional experience in this story of his love affair with Lois. She required his almost constant attention and care during the last years of their life together, and I can almost hear some of their friends characterizing Ed as "a saint" during this period.

But, surely, as we find in his own words, Ed would not have so characterized his role during that long period of Lois's infirmity. With all the love within him, he was simply extending to the inevitable end his moments with his beloved.

Lois died, and we must feel that Ed prolonged their closeness by putting their love on paper. And then Ed rejoined Lois.

Walter Cronkite

PROLOGUE

Lois suspected it was Alzheimer's disease, and doctors confirmed her suspicion. Month by month, year by year, she would be stripped of her powers; perhaps she would die a stranger.

Lois was my wife. She was stricken by the disease along with 4 million other Americans, translating into heartache for tens of millions of family members. Some patients succumb sweetly; others are cruelly transformed. For them, loss of memory is the least consequence of the disease; their very essence is gone.

Despite progress in research, Alzheimer's disease rages out of control. Because Americans are living longer, the number of diagnosed victims is growing at the rate of 1,000 per day. Estimates predict there will be 15 million Alzheimer's patients in the United States by the year 2050; almost four times the number of patients there are today.

This book is a small memorial to my Lois. It is also a case history. I hope that by telling Lois's story in intimate detail, sparing neither of us, I may not only contribute in some way to the understanding of this foul disease, but also provide a measure of comfort for others—for I found comfort at the end.

FOR LOVE OF LOIS

1995–1996

It came slowly, sneakily, so I don't have a date, but sometime in early 1995, as we walked, Lois kept taking my arm. Evidence, I thought, of her love. Then she began going to bed earlier. For years, watching *Masterpiece Theater* together had been a Sunday-night habit for us, but now she began excusing herself to go to bed. "I'm tired," she would say. I thought this would change, but she kept going to bed early and I was left watching television by myself.

Lois loved to read, usually two books at a time. I remember her reading both McCullough's biography of Truman and a Dick Francis thriller—dessert, she called it—in the same week. But around the time she started going to bed earlier, she also began reading more slowly, an index finger moving along each line, pausing at a word now and then in the same way as a child learning to read.

1

"Honey," I asked, "why are you doing that?" She said it was so that when I spoke, interrupting her reading, she wouldn't lose her place. But it was more that she was having trouble reading. She knew it.

Late in 1995 she got new glasses, but they were no help. Believing—or perhaps hoping—that a mistake had been made, she went back to the optometrist. He checked the lenses against the prescription. "They're fine," he said. He sprayed the glasses with lens cleaner and placed them back on her nose. I now think that, from his manner, he suspected what was wrong. He had seen this happen before.

I realize now that as early as a year before she was diagnosed, Lois knew. As someone who had always followed developments in medicine, she recognized the symptoms and, confiding in no one, set herself a goal: she might ultimately have to go to the infirmary, but she would damn well do everything in her power to put off that day.

Lois was, as our daughter Anne once said, a planner. She planned our move into Goodwin House, the life-care retirement center in Alexandria, Virginia, where we now had lived happily for seven years. We had no hint of Alzheimer's disease when we moved there; it was simply Lois planning in our mid-seventies for whatever might happen. We had been living in retirement in Newburyport, Massachusetts, when she said, "You know, one of us might have a stroke or something, and Anne would have to keep flying up here from Washington. Let's see about a place down there." I hated to leave our home and all our friends, but Lois made sense; we moved to Goodwin House.

So, true to her planning nature Lois began, for the first time, walking for exercise in the hall of our building—twice the whole length of the building and around the corner, up and down the East Wing. She did this faithfully every night. Sometimes I joined her; I wish now I always had. She was no longer up to working out in the exercise class she had attended every weekday since entering Goodwin House, but she got hold of a recording of the class in session and worked with it in our apartment. A piece of music the class danced to was on the tape. One of my most cherished memories of Lois is of her dancing a little dance to that music in the middle of our living room: the dainty steps she took and the serious expression on her face.

I saw nothing ominous in this new exercise plan. I was proud of her for sticking to such a diligent program. But then she said something that puzzled me: "I think it would be good to move to an apartment with two bathrooms." We were in a comfortable two-room apartment with a fine view of the Washington Monument and we had experienced no difficulty with only one bathroom. When I pressed her for a reason for switching to two bathrooms, she said, "I think you would enjoy having one of your own."

We did move into another apartment. Not long afterwards Lois took action that should have alerted me that something was wrong. She bought a plastic chair for the bathtub, although she seemed to have no need for it, and arms for the john, which stood higher than the one in our old apartment and so was easier to get on and off—she had thought of that, too. "Good gosh," I said, "you're not an invalid." She responded that they weren't bad things to have. Her own special bathroom, combined with the strategy she had drawn up for gaining strength through exercise, was part of her plan through which she hoped to stay in the apartment as long as possible.

3

Lois had not picked up a book for a long time when she tried rereading John Hersey's *A Single Pebble*. She read so slowly, so painfully, that I finally became anxious. Checking after she went to bed, I found that after two nights of reading she had progressed no farther in the love story than page four.

It was then, sometime in February 1996, that Lois stopped trying to read and told me: "I do believe I have Alzheimer's." She said it the way she might say, "I think I'll buy a new dress." She didn't say how she came by her belief, nor did I ask. I just put my arms around her.

Lois's strong suspicion that she had Alzheimer's was confirmed on June 17, 1996. On that day, after a series of tests had been carried out, neurologist Stuart Stark gave his diagnosis: "Early mild senile dementia of the Alzheimer's type." That is, not only had Lois's brain undergone the normal degeneration of cells associated with old age—she was now eighty-five—but she also displayed the symptoms of Alzheimer's disease, such as difficulty in recalling recent events. I bridled at the word *senile,* even though it was called mild. It didn't fit Lois: only a few months earlier she had put together—perfectly, the accountant said—the figures for our income tax.

Dr. Stark told us that substantial progress was being made in the battle against Alzheimer's. Much research was being carried out, and he wondered if Lois would participate in a study he was undertaking. Immediately, she said she would. She had always been interested in medicine—I teased her that she should have married a doctor—and now, because of this experiment, her illness would serve a purpose.

Dr. Stark was testing the effects of Cognex, a drug that in some cases has slowed down the progress of the disease. He said he would like to try Cognex with Lois, emphasizing that it was not a cure. She was to take one capsule (10 milligrams) four times a day, one with each meal and the fourth at bedtime. He ordered blood tests to be carried out every two weeks for a month, and then once a month, to check for side effects.

Lois's participation in the drug experiment lasted four days. The first day's dosage subjected her to a savage attack of vomiting. She had not been in bed an hour when the rush came, drenching her and the bedcovers. We had barely cleaned up before another outpouring occurred. This time we caught the mess in a dishpan. Then a few minutes later, yet more vomiting. When Lois had no food to bring up, she retched. It went on through the night, tearing her so that I expected to see blood.

As soon as I thought Dr. Stark would be in his office the next day, I called him. "Let's give her a rest," he said, "then try again in two days."

I wrote to Lois's sister, Jo, in High Point, North Carolina: "Lois is trying a drug that may help. It causes nausea, but she is game and giving it a good try." Then I said, "I must tell you something. It happened after the neurologist had, in effect, told Lois she was terminally ill. We had gone to bed. I was lying awake when, from her bed, she said, 'Don't worry.' I assumed she was referring to her illness. But it wasn't that. She reached out in the darkness and took my hand and said, 'I *know* the book will be published. It's the best writing you ever did.' My God, she had been thinking not of her death sentence, but of me and my book!"

Lois did try the drug again, one capsule after each meal, another when she went to bed. The result was another night as terrible as the first. Toward morning, after she had been retching for hours, Lois told me determinedly she would not take

5

the drug anymore, and I said, "Yes, honey, no more." When I told Dr. Stark, he didn't try to change our minds. Nor did he suggest experimentation with another drug.

Lois was not lacking in courage: in addition to her openness to the drug experiment, there was a remarkable letter she sent to her sister in November 1996. The Mack to whom Lois refers in the letter is her ninety-three-year-old brother, and Juanita her deceased sister. Alison and Lisa are our granddaughters, Rob is their father, and Diana their stepmother; their mother, our younger daughter, Lois, died of a brain aneurysm when she was thirty-three. The Anne she refers to is our other daughter, who, with her love and expertise as a nurse, sustained us.

Lois's words—the malformed scattered among the well-formed—betray her illness. But I am proud of the *character* they reveal. The letter prompts the "maudlin tears" that the British scholar C. S. Lewis says he shed after his own wife's death.

We did not see Dr. Stark again. Dr. Robert Heinen, a tall, softly spoken Minnesotan, had been our primary physician since we had moved to Goodwin House. It was he who managed Lois's case expertly, with gentleness, to the end.

November 15, 1996

Dear Josephine,
          I have delayed
too long writing my
sad news to you. I
about two months
ago I had trouble walking
and then I had trouble
talking. By then the
Doctors had decided
it was Alzheimer's—
or what Juanita had
except the Dr. called
hers Senile Dimentia.
So I guess I'm in for
a good long siege, but
I will be taken good
care of. Don't worry.

I haven't written Mack.
I think he has
too much trouble
of his own to worry
about mine.

It had to be
something — so
now I know what.
It is hard on Ed, who
is having a bout of
real bad Rheumatoid
arthritis —

I'm sorry that I
won't be able to go
to alison's wedding
in the spring. She
has brought her husband —
to be to see us twice
and we love him. They

will live near Rob
and Diana in Conn.
Lisa will come home
from Italy for the
Wedding. Anne will
see that Ed gets there.
I hope your large family
is well, all of the
grown-ups and all
the babies — I wish I
could see all of them.
Keep in touch with
Ed and Anne. They
love you and so do
I.
Don't be too sad —
I'm not!
Lois

1997

Lois was using a walker now. It had been a year since Dr. Stark had given his diagnosis, and Lois had become dangerously unsteady. The therapist gave her a simple walker with no receptacle or seat. It did have, curiously, a tennis ball on the foot of each back leg: an improvisation, I was told, to keep the walker from sliding. Lois accepted the walker, showing no embarrassment that it announced her disability. But she could not manage it: she could not walk down a hallway without colliding first into one wall, then the other. I couldn't believe it. At fourteen Lois had been driving her father's Model-T. She had driven cars for seventy years, yet now she could not steer a walker.

Because I couldn't believe this transformation, or didn't want to believe it, I was impatient with Lois: "Just steer down the middle," I would say firmly. *"Down the middle."* I would point the walker toward the middle of the hallway, and she would take perhaps five steps before again ramming a wall. Then, once more, I'd set her on course and repeat, *"In the middle."* It was sad she had come to that—and sad I couldn't have been more understanding.

One day, in an assertion of independence, she left the apartment without her walker—not once, but three times. I came back from shopping and found a note on the floor just inside the door where I couldn't miss it.

Honey, I've gone to eat. I'll also get mail. It wasn't up when I first went down.

This was the last of hundreds, possibly thousands, of notes we exchanged over the years. They began in 1943 when I was working the 5 P.M. to 1 A.M. shift at CBS News, first as writer, then as night editor. Arriving home, I'd find a note from Lois on the kitchen table telling me how her evening had been, news such as "Anne's cold seems better" or "Jo called tonight." Before going to bed, I would write a note to her—on the pad we kept handy for just this purpose—about my night at work. Six of her notes have survived, two of which are shown here. The first is self-explanatory.

The second refers, most likely, to the ten-minute newscast I was writing at that time.

When I was out of town on assignment, or later when I did consulting at television stations around the country, I could count on finding a note from Lois when I opened my suitcase. This is the only one that survives:

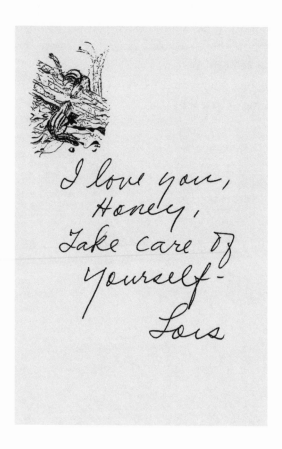

I love you, Honey, Take care of yourself —
Lois

Throughout our sixty years together we were sweethearts.

Our engagement calendar shows that Lois was still getting out early in 1997, despite her difficulties with the walker. I find a notation: "Last shopping together, Lord & Taylor, January 11." We had gone to the Western Avenue store in Washington, D.C. I don't remember what either of us bought, but I do remember that when we arrived home she took from her purse two tiny vials of Chanel cologne—samples, she said, I might like to have "sometime when you're putting on the dog." I never got around to using them while she lived, and they still sit with a scattering of cough drops on a tray in my bathroom. I may sprinkle myself with this cologne some day, but that will have to be for an occasion I cannot imagine.

The entry for March 8 reads "Anne took Lois shopping," and two weeks later the calendar shows I took her to the dentist. Every other Tuesday, nurses checked Lois's blood pressure. She still went for her routine Friday shampoos in the Goodwin House beauty shop at that time, and Anne washed Lois's hair when she visited on Tuesdays; I could tell when Anne had set Lois's hair because of the lovely waves she made in it. We still attended concerts in the auditorium, ate dinner with friends, and watched Mark Russell in his *Comedy Specials* on television. Lois laughed with him as easily as ever. It was almost as though the disease had paused to reconsider taking hold.

But then came April 21—Lois broke her arm. I was with her when she fell. She was getting up from a nap, and even now as I write I hear the arm breaking. It sounded like the splintering of a dead branch. I placed a pillow under her head and told her not to move. To myself I said, "This isn't happening."

I telephoned the Goodwin House clinic and the nurse called for an ambulance. The ambulance seemed a long time coming. When I checked out in the hall for the ambulance crew, so help me, a woman going by called out in greeting, "Oh, happy day!" The ambulance came soon after that.

At the hospital the emergency room was in its typical, busy state. In due course, a nurse took Lois's temperature and listened to her heart. Laboratory technicians made an electrocardiograph and took blood. X-rays were taken of her arm, and a doctor reported, "She has a fracture of the humerus." I was glad it was the left arm. Lois, waiting in her cubicle, said little. We held hands.

Lois was admitted to the hospital on Dr. Heinen's orders. I went with her to her room. I can't remember what we said, but I know when I kissed her and said goodnight she smiled. It was just like the reassurance she had given me the night our second child was born: that night on the steps of the hospital, she had smiled and said, "Everything's going to be all right." Now, years later, *she* was again reassuring *me*.

Dr. Heinen kept Lois in the hospital another night. When she came home she was put in Room 229 on the second floor, which serves as our infirmary—a place where residents of Goodwin House recover from surgery as well as illness, and where the terminally ill die. I had hoped Lois could be with me. Instead, she would be kept on the second floor for two months.

As John Bayley said of his wife, novelist Iris Murdoch, Alzheimer's patients are not always gentle. One morning in the infirmary, in a rage born of frustration, Lois threw a glassful of water into the face of an aide. I was there and saw it and could not believe gentle Lois was doing that. I was scared. I knew that some Alzheimer's patients undergo a complete change in personality. Sweet people turn sour; sometimes terribly ugly. Was this the start of that?

Anne, my dearest RN, tried to allay my fear. The change, she said, might be due not just to progress of the disease, but also to a reaction between the painkillers for her broken arm and medication related to Alzheimer's disease. The day after I had this conversation with Anne, Dr. Heinen told me that, while Lois was in the hospital and being closely monitored, he had prescribed Aricept, a new drug designed to alleviate the symptoms of Alzheimer's disease. "Perhaps," he said, "I shouldn't have tried that." I respect him for telling me—he didn't have to.

I was visiting with Lois in the infirmary one morning when a psychiatrist appeared. She introduced herself as Stephanie Heidelberg. My reaction was, what's a psychiatrist doing here? But Dr. Heidelberg had not come to put Lois on the couch; she had come to examine her and prescribe medication for her behavioral disorder. In a test of memory, Lois gave her birth date correctly as July 16. When Dr. Heidelberg asked her what year, she began, "Nineteen—," paused, then repeated, "Nineteen." Dr. Heidelberg said quickly, "So it was 1919." I don't think Lois meant 1919; I think she was making another try for 1911 and was cut off.

When Lois began crying, Dr. Heidelberg asked me if that happened often. I said, "Fairly often," and she said she would prescribe Zoloft, an antidepressant. I never again saw Lois behave violently, but often she would go into a terrible crying spell that no amount of hugging and beseeching could stop.

"Don't let it bother you," the nurses said. "Her threshold for crying is way low." They were saying she couldn't help it because of brain damage, but I was not comforted. For such piteous crying there had to be huge frustration. Fortunately—and I thanked God for it—she had peaceful days, too.

A trivial problem, by comparison, was her roommate's addiction to television. Her set blasted from breakfast to bedtime, making conversation with Lois almost impossible. Whenever I asked this woman if I could turn down the volume, she was all sweetness: "Yes, of course." But as soon as I left her, she sent it roaring back up. The nurses had no more success, and nothing was done. I suppose, like me, they didn't want a fuss.

This woman also had a habit that was revolting. She would often pull up her nightgown and, in police parlance, expose herself. Not only this, but she was continually dabbing herself with tissue and dropping the tissue on the floor. I had to pass her to get to the door, and she often pleaded with me as I tried to get by: "Please pick it up," she would say. "*Please.*" And I would pick it up. I suppose I felt sorry for her.

Lois was not confined to this room. Twice a day, aides set her in a chair in the hallway where she and other patients similarly seated could get a change of scenery. Sitting there in the late afternoon and early evening, they could watch videotapes of old movies starring Judy Garland and Shirley Temple. Or, they would watch one of Lois's favorites, Lawrence Welk's orchestra playing the romantic music of the 1930s and 1940s.

Not long after Lois's arm was set I began taking her to therapy, located temporarily on the ninth floor. There, Lois's arm was manipulated for an hour by a pleasant young therapist named Melanie, who managed, in a most gentle way, to give Lois a thorough workout. I didn't stay for the whole hour, but came back when the time was up. Now I wonder how I could have done that.

At about this same time, I started bringing Lois up to our apartment to see the soap opera *As the World Turns*. It is the only "soap" she ever watched, and I think that she watched it now out of nostalgia as much as anything. It was nostalgia for the happy time, years earlier, when she had first started watching it: our younger daughter had not died, and we were living in Dobbs Ferry, a cozy village on the Hudson, all of us together with our tiger-striped cat, Scamper.

Lois was well enough in May for me to take her to the main dining room for dinner. She had no difficulty in feeding herself or carrying on conversation.

I have also discovered how serviceably Lois wrote at that stage. She had an appointment with a podiatrist on May 19, and I find this sample of her handwriting in the calendar:

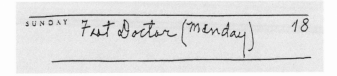

Her handwriting had deteriorated—the *o* in Monday was an *a*—but she had her wits.

Then came a Sunday when, with permission, I brought her to the apartment for a meal of diced chicken, stir-fried with crushed red peppers and mushrooms. I did not know it, but this was the first of dozens of stir-fry suppers I would fix for us on Sunday evenings. The only difference was that later Lois drank buttermilk instead of tea, and we often had rice. Another part of our Sunday-evening tradition was sherry. Lois was fond of sherry—she liked it with ice, which I thought abominable—and for a long time, until she had trouble swallowing, I kept a bottle of Harvey's Bristol Cream handy for her to enjoy.

A big disappointment that May of 1997 was Lois's inability to attend the wedding of our granddaughter Alison in Connecticut. I am sure I was a poor substitute for "Lady," whom Alison adored. But we had good news in June when Dr. Heinen declared Lois fit to return to the apartment, to return to me. What a privilege it was to look across the room any time of day and see her; to watch Dan Rather and the evening news with her; to hug her any time I felt like it; to tease and kiss her; and at bedtime, to pray with her. When praying, we often recited together the verse written long ago by John Charles McNeill, who was a friend of Lois's father and poet laureate of North Carolina:

> Dear Lord, we know so little what is best
> Wingless, we move so lowly,
> But in Thy all-knowledge let us rest,
> O holy, holy, holy.

I knew our reunion was temporary, that I could not have her like this for long. But the preciousness of the moment, the gift, made for gratitude. It produced, along with sadness, a deeper appreciation. Of her, of love, of life.

She was back with me only eleven days before her blood pressure soared to 210 over 100, and Dr. Heinen ordered her back to the second floor for monitoring. The next day the pressure was down to 160 over 80, and soon she was back with me in the apartment. Thanks to medication, Lois was doing well. Records show that at this time—early June 1997—she was receiving 180 mg of Cardizem for her heart, 50 mg of Cozaar for her high blood pressure, 0.1 mg of Synthroid as a thyroid supplement, and 500 mg of Tylenol for back pain caused by a fall. Except for the Tylenol, she was taking these medications once a day. I saw no mention of Zoloft on the list, although I have no doubt it was administered at times.

On July 28, 1997, this note of appreciation written by Lois appeared in the *Gazette*, Goodwin House's weekly newsletter: "A heartfelt thank-you to the dear people who, through flowers, notes, and prayers, helped me in my difficult time of tumbles. Truly, friends like you are a blessing. Lois Bliss." All our married life, Lois had been the one who wrote the required letters of congratulation and sympathy, and always in a kinder, more original way than I ever could. My only contribution in this instance had been to place the hyphen in *thank-you*. What she wrote may have been a scribble, but in expression she had not lost her touch. Good phrase, that "difficult time of tumbles."

Lois was, in fact, still writing a few brief letters. When she found she could no longer write without the sentences giving the impression of roller coasters, she took a sheet of paper and, with a ruler and black marker, composed a page of bold parallel lines. For a while she wrote on pages placed over these lines that showed through and served as a guide. But when Lois found herself unable to assemble properly the letters to form words, she wrote a final loving letter to Lisa, the first grandchild to make "Lady" their name for her, and gave up.

I know precisely the last time she legibly wrote her name. It was in the forenoon of October 22, 1997. She was signing a paper designating Anne as the one to decide whether life-prolonging procedures should be withheld. Anne and I had discussed this. Lois had often said she did not want merely to live, to be a vegetable, and I had said that while Lois's wish should be respected, it would be a terribly painful decision for me to make. Anne, sparing me, said she would decide. I watched sadly as Lois, who as a schoolgirl had excelled in penmanship, wrote her name with immense effort:

I feel a sense of shame for showing, as it were, this wound of hers. At the same time, I take pride in Lois's endeavor. My sweetheart took care to dot the *i*'s and cross both *t*'s and, bless her, if you look closely, you will see she placed a period at the end.

Lois was failing in all kinds of ways. She could no longer do laundry: the dials confused her, and lifting clothes out of the washer hurt her back. But when I went to the laundry room to do washing, she would come anyway, and because she wanted so desperately to help, I asked her if she would measure out the detergent. "You know best," I said, "how much we need." I doubt she was deceived.

A symptom that took me by surprise was her difficulty in making simple decisions. I first noticed this when, going through the cafeteria line, it became almost impossible for her to decide which entree she wanted. Her indecision caused delay for those in line behind us, and was embarrassing. When I reported this to Anne, she told me to decide for Lois. I did, but hated to. It was another score for Alzheimer's.

She no longer tried to cook, but a tiny wooden duck inscribed "Lois's Kitchen" hung—still hangs—on the wall beside our stove. Lois enjoyed cooking, but it was something in which she had virtually no experience when we married, for she had gone directly from college to teach at the State School for the Blind in Raleigh, where she ate in the school's dining room. I believe *The Boston Cook Book* was the first book she bought when we set up housekeeping. Following directions, she became a fine cook and kept on defiantly until the spring of 1997. The last dish she prepared was a tomato salad to take to Anne and her husband, Tom. Whenever we went for a meal in their home in Washington, D.C., a fine salad was her contribution.

There were several occasions when, watching television, we caught a discussion of Alzheimer's disease, its treatment, and prospects for a cure. We heard the English critic John Bayley talk about his wife Iris's experience with the disease, and Lois listened with great interest. So, although we did not seek out these programs, we never turned away. From the beginning we had the attitude: Let's take this thing head-on. But then one afternoon in late 1997, listening to a panel discussion of Alzheimer's, Lois appeared uneasy. She was not looking at the television set but around the room.

"Honey," I said, "do you want to hear any more programs like this?"

"No," she said, and that was the last one.

It was in the summer of 1997 that I started keeping a diary. What was happening was so momentous that I wrote less from desire than from demand. *I had to do it.* What follows here are passages from the diary; these are the words that convey most truthfully and candidly the events, and emotions, from that difficult time. I also include additional notes, written now, with Lois no longer here, in my attempt to describe my sweetheart and her brave battle.

I think of Lois as being about as perfect as anyone can be. She was capable, loyal, and loving, and there is no way I can make anyone who did not know my dearest comrade know her truly. I think of the frustration John Bayley experienced: "The Iris of my words cannot be any Iris who existed"—so true of my words and my Lois.

I began the diary with an accident.

JULY 8: Lois fell. Nothing broken, but she strained her neck. She was in the bedroom, just walking, and fell.

JULY 9: Am massaging her neck with old-fashioned Bengay. She sits in a straight chair, and I stand behind her and massage. I take pleasure in this, not only from helping her, but from a sense of intimacy.

JULY 12: No more massaging. The neck's OK.

JULY 16: Lois's birthday. Our next-door neighbor Barbara Bishop organized a small dinner party.

Twelve friends attended the dinner. Lois turned eighty-six. There was a cake with a lighted candle that Lois put out with one good blow. It was her last real party. Lois liked Barbara, a

most cheerful, helpful person who, although American, once
served as an Anglican nun in England.

JULY 18: They have changed Lois's medication again.
Besides 50 mg of Zoloft (the antidepressant) at bedtime,
she's also getting 25 mg at 9 A.M. and 1 P.M. I am struck
by how she cries, but in conversation she is composed.

JULY 19: This evening looking out at a full moon, Lois
whispered, "Beautiful." One word.

JULY 20: In many ways, Lois's mind is sharp. She knows
her affliction, recognizes people, remembers who is
writing to her, and can do arithmetic even though she
can't write. Yesterday a fellow resident, Helen
Fredlund, who volunteers at the Washington National
Cathedral and knows that Lois once taught blind
children, asked if Lois could do Braille. She still can,
and so, someday in that great cathedral, people will
kneel on a cushion needle-pointed with the words
"God is love" in the language of the blind.

Three or four weeks ago I told Lois I didn't like the
way I was ending my father's biography, which I have
been working on for some time, in such a routine
way—with his death. Without hesitation she said,
"Why don't you end it with rinderpest, and how far
they've come in trying to eradicate it? Father fought it
so." A century ago rinderpest was the most deadly
cattle disease in Africa and Asia. In one year it destroyed
half the water buffalo population of the Philippines. As

a medical missionary in China, my father tried to develop a serum for rinderpest. So the book will end, as Lois suggested, with the United Nations Food and Agriculture Organization's prediction that, due to new treatment and improved early detection, eradication of the plague is possible by 2010. Lois is still my editor.

JULY 21: I asked Lois if she would sew on a button for me. She did, but with such difficulty I won't ask again.

JULY 25: I'm now reading poetry to Lois from a little book, *Songs Merry and Sad*, written by Lois's father's friend John Charles McNeill. Her favorite is the poem "When I Go Home." It starts:

When I go home, green, green will grow the grass,
Whereon the flight of sun and cloud will pass.
Long lines of wood-ducks through the deepening gloam
Will hold above the West, as wrought on brass
And fragrant furrows will have delved the loam
When I go home.

After two more stanzas, the poem ends with the line, "And, oh, 'twill be a day to rest and roam when I go home." Lois enjoys this because of the lovely sound of the words.

Until Lois became ill we read almost no poetry together. The only poem I remember sharing was one of Edgar Allan Poe's, which, because of the wording, I recited when we were in bed and I was lying by her side:

Now all the nighttide I lie by the side
Of my darling, my wife and my bride
In the sepulcher by the sea,
In the tomb by the sounding sea.

In that other time, long ago, we were charmed and haunted by these lines. With Lois dying, I could not recite them—though I was tempted.

I recall a time when Lois and I lay side-by-side before we were married. This happened on a weekend in June 1940. Lois was vacationing with her mother at Carolina Beach. I was working at the *Citizen*, the Scripps Howard paper in Columbus, Ohio: a good newspaper doomed to die, like so many other afternoon papers, at the hands of television's evening news. I had just bought a secondhand Ford and decided, on a Saturday, to drive overnight to North Carolina, see Lois, and return in time for work on Monday.

I cut down through West Virginia and reached the beach Sunday afternoon. Lois had no idea I was coming, so surprising her made a great moment. I remember we took a walk on the beach. Afterward I slept, and when I awoke, Lois was lying beside me. It meant a great deal to me that she did that. After supper, I started the long drive back to Columbus. Buoyant. Full of confidence in our forthcoming marriage.

JULY 27: Lunch with Bill and Helen Roberts at the Peking Gourmet Inn. Lois ordered her favorite dishes: tofu and hot and sour soup.

Bill, retired, had served as assistant press secretary to President Ford and as chairman to the Radio-Television News Directors

Association (RTNDA). We had become friendly with Bill and Helen at RTNDA meetings. Bill died not long before Lois. A journalist and a gentleman.

JULY 28: Lois was discharged from therapy. Has good use of the arm broken in April.

AUGUST 1: My sweetheart looked lovely this morning. Sitting beside her as she finished breakfast, I said, "I'd like to run off and marry you." Then, clear as can be, she said, "Then why don't you?"

AUGUST 2: Lois's support of me in what I attempt is incredible. This morning I was leaving to mail to a prospective publisher a little book I had written about my boyhood in China. She blessed it. She touched the envelope and said, "God bless it, and God bless you, too." That's what she has been like all the way. No wonder I love her.

When I think what a comrade Lois was, how dear and devoted she always managed to be, I often think of how, in a surprising way, she supported me in 1993. I was to receive a national award.* Walter Cronkite was to present it, and I would have the opportunity to preach the gospel of Edward R. Murrow to more than one thousand broadcast journalists assembled in the grand ballroom of the Fontainebleau Hotel in Miami Beach. Without doubt, it would be the most important speech

---

*The Paul White Award, presented annually by the RTNDA.

of my career, and for the journalists, the subject most vital: the standards for what we do.

A week before the meeting I developed pleurisy. It became increasingly painful, and Lois urged me to see Dr. Heinen. She told me, "Don't wait." I told her I had to wait; Dr. Heinen would put me in the hospital and I would miss this crowning moment. When she persisted, I said I didn't care if it killed me; I had to make the speech. I meant it. She knew I meant it and knew what the speech meant to me, and said nothing more.

I gave the speech. I went to Dr. Heinen as soon as I returned and was hospitalized for twelve days. On the first day they shot me with morphine: I had gone screaming down the hall in pain.

I don't know how many wives, loving their husbands, would act as Lois had. I suppose she stopped her urging in part because it was useless and because she knew few people die of pleurisy. But I believe a big part of it was that, understanding my passion to make the speech, she was with me.

AUGUST 4: A family reunion. Lisa, back from Italy, and
  Alison and her husband, Wayne, down from
  Connecticut, here for a two-day visit.

Since college, Lisa had been working for a marketing firm in Milan.

AUGUST 6: Shopped at Sears. Lois went along but stayed
  in the car.

AUGUST 26: Our fifty-seventh wedding anniversary. I laid
  on a Lincoln town car, with driver, for a candlelight

dinner at the Mount Vernon Inn. The drive down along the Potomac at sunset was a dream. So was the whole evening. We had a cozy corner table, champagne, great food, and the limo waiting for us when we were done.

I'm so glad, and grateful, that we did this. Another year and it would have been impossible.

SEPTEMBER 8: Lois, holding tightly to my arm, took a long walk in the garden. When we came to the North Woods where I thought, being tired, she would want to turn back, she said, "Let's go see the hydrangea." She was pleased to see the plant doing nicely.

Anne and Tom had given us the hydrangea at Easter. We had it on our coffee table and then, after a few weeks, I planted it in the North Woods. The North and South Woods are behind our building. Each consists of about two hundred trees— maples and oaks mostly—so these woods are small. They are full of wildflowers and daffodils planted by generations of residents. A year after this "long walk"—our last walk because Lois would soon need a wheelchair—a bulldozer carried off our hydrangea for no good reason. I told Lois what had happened, and wish I hadn't.

Paths run through both the North and South woods, and here and there beside the paths are benches. It was before planting the hydrangea that Lois and I had settled upon a bench in the South Woods; for the next three years—as long as Lois lived—we regarded it as "our" bench. We were there together, visiting to the accompaniment of bird songs every afternoon the weather allowed it.

SEPTEMBER 13: For the first time in two months, Lois
went down to the dining room for lunch *and* dinner. In
the afternoon, with the help of her walker, she went to
her garden box to see how the mint was doing.

OCTOBER 5: Granddaughter Alison and Wayne Amente,
married five months, have come down from
Connecticut to visit. Last night we all had dinner at
Anne and Tom's. Great grilled hamburgers by Tom.
This morning Alison and Wayne came over here and
we had a precious time. Both Lois and I think Wayne,
who is manager of a post office in Connecticut—
Darien, I believe—is splendid. They appear very much
in love.

OCTOBER 18: I'm so glad for that bench in the South
Woods. We sit there so often that other people leave it
for us. It's there I read Lois the mail. She listens and, I
believe, understands everything.

A piece of mail that came each week was the Order of Wor-
ship for services at our church in Newburyport. It includes a
paragraph—always the same—that everyone in the church
reads aloud before leaving. It begins, "Go now in peace, never
be afraid," and ends, "Go now in peace, in faith, and in love."
I didn't read it to Lois every week, but when I did she listened
with full attention, gaining strength from it, as I did.

OCTOBER 29: Took Lois to a band concert in the
auditorium. It's endearing the way she applauds after
each number, hands scarcely touching.

OCTOBER 30: We attended a regional RTNDA luncheon at George Washington University. We have attended dozens of RTNDA meetings together, and I can't help wondering if we shall attend another.

OCTOBER 31: A letter today from a friend, Colonel Arthur "Barney" Oldfield, USAF, retired, whose wife Vada fought Alzheimer's disease with something approaching ferocity for eleven years. He wrote, "In my thoughts, I go side by side with you." Kind of him to write.

NOVEMBER 9: Lois no longer interested in her soap opera. Tom gave us tapes of books to play. Just the thing, I thought, but, to my surprise, Lois won't listen.

NOVEMBER 16: About that prayer of ours, "God is great, God is good, and we thank him for this day." I improvised last night, adding "and for our love that stays in bloom." A bit overwrought, Lois thought.

NOVEMBER 17: I went to a conference sponsored by the Northern Virginia Chapter of the Alzheimer's Association and came away with good instruction by the keynote speaker, Lela Knox Shanks, whose husband recently died of the disease. She spoke of "hidden treasures" in the experience, calling it "the most difficult but most rewarding of my life." The greatest gift, she said, was the discovery of unconditional love. "I found that I could love more than I had ever loved before." Glad I went.

DECEMBER 2: The popular pianist John Eaton performed tonight, and Lois and I enjoyed him as usual. Eaton's first piano teacher, now deceased, was a resident of Goodwin House. He used to come to play for her, and still comes periodically. He favors composers such as George Gershwin and Richard Rodgers, so, naturally, with us old folks he's a hit. I notice that, despite her illness, Lois still applauds.

DECEMBER 10: Bill and Jeanne Hamilton had us up to their apartment for drinks, then dinner downstairs. A retired Foreign Service officer, Bill had important posts in Thailand and other parts of Southeast Asia. Lois requested sherry. I tattled on her: I told the story of how once at a cocktail party, Lois had told me she wanted a Virgin Mary. Before I could get it, Bill Moyers had asked if he could bring her something from the bar, and Lois asked for white wine. When Moyers left to get the wine, I said, "But, honey, you wanted a Virgin Mary." "I know," she said, "but how could I say *virgin* to Bill Moyers?"

That time at the Hamiltons' was the last time Lois went to someone else's place for drinks. And now, five years later, it is sweet Jeanne who is struck by Alzheimer's.

DECEMBER 25: As usual we had Christmas with Anne's family in Washington, D.C. Lois was in good spirits. At dinner our grandson Andrew sat next to her and helped cut her meat. I like Andrew. He is very gentle and loving with Lois.

Before going over to Anne's, Lois opened my gifts: some Chanel No. 5—the kind you spray—and a blouse. She gave me a wallet of the finest leather I've ever seen. Ever felt. I told her there was still wear in the wallet I had, but I would treasure hers and use it proudly one day. Why did I have to tell her that? She was so happy to have it to give to me.

By the next Christmas Lois was too weak for Anne, or anyone else, to take her shopping. "I'm sorry," she said, "I have nothing to give you." I told her, "Oh, yes, you do," and showed her the wallet she had given me and I hadn't used. I tried hard to make her see that this really was a new gift; one that, starting that day, I was going to enjoy. I still use it. I hate to think of it wearing out—dread any sign of that.

Lois had a way of choosing marvelous gifts, the fine billfold being the most ordinary. Guarding the entrance to our apartment, over in the corner from where I write, stands what pretends to be a lion from the Ming Tombs, only he is plaster of Paris. Lois gave him to me more than forty years ago either for Christmas or my birthday. I don't remember which.

I am also using a key ring she gave me. Such an everyday item, you say. Ah, but this key ring is a miniature Chinese lock, one with a sliding bolt. I never asked where she found it. Another special gift from Lois conceals the littered bottom shelf below our television. It is an original Japanese store sign bearing large characters on sandalwood. I have no idea what the characters are saying, but I know the love that Lois was expressing when she gave it to me.

1998

JANUARY 3: Took Lois to a concert tonight. Really good
choral group, maybe thirty male voices. My lady had a
good time, and so did I. We were together.

JANUARY 4: Jo called. Lois listens to her sister most
seriously, as though memorizing the words to keep as
treasure. She may wonder if she will hear Jo's voice
again.

Lois had three sisters and a brother, and by this time her brother, Mack, and two sisters Juanita and Odessa had died; Jo was
the only one left.

There is a story in Mack. From early boyhood he had loved
baseball, and as a college student he pitched for Wake Forest.

He wanted to turn pro but his father told him to aim higher, so he earned a degree in law. But he never practiced. His father died, freeing him from "higher aims," and he had a successful career playing for minor league teams all over the South.

When Mack retired from baseball and joined the sales staff of WWNC radio station in Asheville, he did not leave baseball; he became a scout for the Baltimore Orioles, checking out high school pitchers in towns all around. He did this until his ninetieth birthday, when he told Oriole management he was too old for driving about in the North Carolina mountains and was quitting.

The Orioles said, "You can't do that to us." They sent an emissary down from Baltimore and signed him, at the age of ninety, to a new five-year contract. The story appeared on sports pages all over the country—almost the whole first page of the sports section in the *Baltimore Sun*—and National Public Radio sent a crew to North Carolina to cover the extraordinary man in action. Mack worked for three years of the contract before he died in 1997. He was a tall, lean man; a fine man, the picture of a pitcher.

I must tell you something about Lois. I was to discover that sporting achievement ran in her family. We had been married a year when I came across her Meredith College yearbook and discovered I'd wed an athlete: she had played first string on the school's basketball team for three years and field hockey all four years. She had served as vice president of the honor society and business manager of the basketball team. She had also reported for the college paper. Not only this, but Lois had borne our first child before I learned from her sisters that she was a direct descendant of George Washington's grandfather,

Colonel Ball. When I asked her why she hadn't told me these things, she made out they weren't important.

FEBRUARY 4: This afternoon as Lois and I were going to get the mail, she suddenly said, "You aren't going to marry one of the women here, are you?" I said, "Not a chance." I wonder if she could have been serious. Perhaps half-serious, some of the Alzheimer's speaking.

FEBRUARY 11: Lois no longer follows me to the laundry room and last week stopped making her bed. The shutdown is terrible to see.

FEBRUARY 13: Took Lois to the Goodwin House beauty shop for her Friday-morning shampoo. Afterward we sat by a window, and the light of the winter sun on her white hair formed a kind of incandescence I can't describe.

FEBRUARY 15: In winter we open our mail in the apartment or the Goodwin House parlor where, in the late afternoon, we are alone. Today we had *two* Newburyport letters and a bank statement.

It's hard for me to see how I could knowingly distress Lois, and do it opening envelopes, but I did. It had been Lois's habit to keep all business correspondence in the envelope it came in, and now she saw me throwing away the envelopes so I'd have room in my crowded files. I could see it hurt her to watch me do it, but I was so convinced of the rightness of what I was doing, the practicality of it, that by God I was going to continue doing it. Now, that look she had on her face haunts me. Her expression was less of disapproval than of injury. I was violating what she thought best, the procedure she had followed all her adult life. A matter of envelopes, a small matter; but if it is small, then why am I crying?

MARCH 4: Lois is so loyal. We were in the solarium—too
   cold for outdoors—and a woman asked how I had
   done in a television interview. Before I could reply Lois
   said, "Well, my husband did wonderfully." And tonight
   when I said, "Now, you have sweet dreams," she said, "I
   know I hope you do." I shake my head.

The interview had been on public television. Elizabeth Farnsworth had interviewed Dan Schorr and me upon the death of Fred Friendly, the legendary documentary producer for whom we both had worked.

MARCH 5: We had dinner tonight with Armisted Lee,
   who was in the Foreign Service, and his wife, Eleanore.
   Lois enjoys them, as do I. Like me, Armie is the son of
   China missionaries. Eleanore, a Vermonter—and proud
   of it—brightens everything with her humor. Because
   the four of us are Democrats, we have a lovely time
   bashing Republicans.

Armie died within the year. He was younger than I am, and I had counted on him being a companion for as long as I was around.

MARCH 8: I feel tonight that I have fallen in love with Lois
   all over again. She is being wonderfully brave.

MARCH 11: Set up house today in Apartment 601, a temporary move from 520 while they put in new windows and air conditioning there. Goodwin House employees used a dolly for the heavy stuff; Lois helped with small things, even though she uses a walker. She wants desperately to help.

MARCH 13: Card dated February 25 received from Cronkite in Vietnam. He says the place is "vastly changed, and the people very friendly." I read the brief message to Lois, making sure she understood the sign-off: "Best to you both." *Both.* Cronkite thinks a lot of Lois. When he gave me an autographed copy of his memoir, *A Reporter's Life,* I noticed he wrote, "and your wonderful wife." Well, he has a wonderful wife, too.

MARCH 19: Lois (me, too) tickled that we now have a great granddaughter. She is Alexandra, eight pounds, fifteen ounces, born to Alison and Wayne. Lovely brown eyes; a siren already.

MARCH 22: ABC News' Jackie Judd, her husband Michael Shulman, and six-year-old twin sons, Philip and Andrew, came to visit. After a good time in the apartment, they took us for dinner at the local Hilton. The boys are bright and extremely well behaved. How Lois enjoyed them! She remembers holding them in her lap when they were babies—an armful.

This was Lois's last meal in a restaurant.

MARCH 24: Today Lois said to me quietly and without difficulty, as though she had rehearsed it, "I am not afraid to die." She was sitting in the Victorian chair, not her rocker, because its seat is higher and easier to get out of. I sense this is something she has been thinking about saying and decided this was the time. She wanted me to know. Saying nothing, I knelt and kissed her.

MARCH 25: She keeps saying things that touch me. When I told her today, "Together, honey, we're going to make it," she said slowly, one separate word at a time, "I wouldn't want to make it (long pause) with anyone but you." No way could I put a price on that.

MARCH 27: News has lost none of its fascination for Lois. David Frost interviewed Cronkite tonight on PBS and I don't think Lois missed a word.

APRIL 1: Today we moved back to Apartment 520. We enjoyed 601. It was a corner apartment with great views and less clutter because we hadn't bothered to bring up the couch and large cabinet. Still, it's good to be back. Fun tonight listening to Mark Russell.

APRIL 3: Lois hasn't lost her knack for finding four-leaf clovers. Out in the garden she looked down and matter-of-factly picked up another for her collection. She keeps more than a dozen of them pressed on heavy paper in a little box.

APRIL 4: The four-leaf clover has brought very bad luck. Getting out of bed this morning, Lois stumbled over a packing box left over from the move and broke her hip. Tonight she is in Alexandria Hospital. What else can happen?

APRIL 5: After a night in the hospital Lois is now being cared for on the second floor. Fortunately she feels no pain. The downside is she may need a wheelchair.

APRIL 7: Lois looks much better; alert. Reminded me that income tax is due.

This was only the fourth year in our long marriage that Lois didn't prepare the returns. In college she had majored in math. She respected numbers. "They never lie," she said.

APRIL 16: We're back together in the apartment. No wheelchair, thank goodness; just the walker. For now, meals are brought to her. Sometimes I bring up my meals so we can eat together.

APRIL 18: Lois showed strange behavior. I returned from dinner to find she had pulled off the elastic hose prescribed for her hip and put on a nightgown over her blouse. The food brought to her was untouched. I should have stayed with her and will do so from now on.

APRIL 19: I haven't told the clinic what happened, and Lois seems fine today, Sunday. Like old times, we watched Charles Osgood's morning program and *Meet the Press*. Lois paid close attention to both programs. I have my fingers crossed.

APRIL 22: Today, for the second day, Lois seemed unnaturally preoccupied with the highboy in our bedroom, going through each drawer over and over for at least an hour. During her searching, she didn't speak. For some reason, perhaps because I was afraid how she would answer, I didn't speak either. There was a wild look on her face.

I began keeping this diary because of the reporter in me and because of our love, but at this point I became uncomfortable. The diary might make a book, and wasn't I cashing in on Lois's misery? I stopped taking notes for more than a week, and then went back to it: I wanted a record in any case, and should a book result, so be it. Perhaps it would help those who, like me, were seeing loved ones taken, in a real sense, piece by piece. Perhaps I could show that, as I was discovering, along with the ugliness there can be beauty.

So I went on.

MAY 2: Watched the Kentucky Derby together in the apartment. Lois's horse, Real Quiet, won. She *took* my dollar!

MAY 6: Lonely in the apartment. Lois is back on the second floor, and there is no question this is for the best as she has become paranoid. A real shock this afternoon when she scribbled, "I'm held as prisoner."

While I stared at what she had written, she snatched the paper from me and wrote, "Beware."

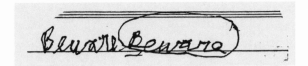

She wrote the word twice, perhaps realizing that the first, poorly written, might not be legible. Then she circled it. This frightens me.

MAY 7: Lois behaved beautifully today. She is on new medication. The wild look has disappeared. No desperate notes; conversation is normal. I am so grateful I could cry.

MAY 8: Good time today. Alison and Wayne came down from Bethel, Connecticut, birthplace of P. T. Barnum, with their firstborn—two-month-old Alexandra. Anne took a wonderful photo of Alexandra in Lois's lap. They look comfy together.

MAY 12: The nurses have observed a return of paranoid behavior, so today it was decided that the psychiatrist should see Lois again and determine what new medication she should take. The decision came at one of the periodic meetings between family and staff.

Dr. Heidelberg did see Lois and again prescribed the antide-pressant Zoloft, and although Lois no longer showed symptoms of paranoia, she still had those terrible sieges of crying. The nurses kept telling me it wasn't as bad as it sounded, that she might cry remembering happy as well as unhappy emotional experiences. But I was not comforted.

MAY 18: When we get the mail—she in a wheelchair now—among the letters we often find magazines, which I give her to hold. In her sloping lap the magazines tend to slide, but with a determination that is touching, she keeps her grasp. I can see that helping in even this small way gives her satisfaction. It is, by God, something she can do.

MAY 24: Today we both signed forms saying that, if in a "terminal condition," we are not to be resuscitated. Her signature was not much more than her "mark."

JUNE 3: Wheeled Lois to her flower box and found the Queen Elizabeth roses doing so well we were able to take a fine bouquet to her room.

JUNE 5: Lois fell out of her wheelchair in our apartment and, because of a communication foul up, had a dickens of a time getting a nurse. Nothing broken, thank goodness. Just this morning I had taken Lois to see Dr. Martinelli, the same bone man who treated her arm. The new x-ray shows the hip has mended nicely. Dr. Martinelli is impressive, both warm and competent. I told him what I thought of him. I felt I could: I'm old and he's young.

1998

JUNE 9: I was at my desk when Lois called, "Honey, full moon!" She was by the window, transfixed by the glorious orange ball on the horizon. It was a sight we often call each other to see. I have a special memory of Lois and the moon. When it was in total eclipse in 1989, Lois, dear heart, was the only resident who watched from our roof garden from beginning to end. It was two in the morning before she came down to bed.

JUNE 10: Out of the blue Lois asked, "Have you done the estimated?" The tax payment is due and I had forgotten. This marvelous woman who has been, in effect, my business manager for half a century hasn't let go.

JUNE 11: On this lovely spring day the Alzheimer's patients and some relatives were taken to a mall, where we had lunch. Lois chose potato salad and Coke, which I could see she enjoyed, along with chocolate ice cream for dessert. Afterward, wheeling Lois about, I came to a men's shop, where I bought a necktie—a Calvin Klein of a solid burgundy color that made it irresistible. Lois saw me pick it out. "Lovely," she said.

That is the last time we were in a shop together. Now when I put on the tie, it's a sad little ceremony.

JUNE 12: They've renewed therapy for Lois's hip. Every time I come by when Lois is receiving treatment, I find

her walking back and forth between parallel bars.
There's padding on the floor in case she falls.

JUNE 15: Today we talked on and on about how we met;
how, in the summer of 1930, she was working as a
waitress at a conference in East Northfield,
Massachusetts; and how, as busboy, I carried her trays.
She said that, coming from North Carolina, she felt she
was in a foreign land in Massachusetts. And, for the
first time, she spoke of the black woman who sat at
one of her tables:
"I had to ask if she wanted coffee, tea, or milk."
"Yes," I said, "and as you asked, you cried."
"Yes."
"But you served her."
She hoped part of why she cried was that she was
ashamed that she found serving the woman so hard. I
told her I was sure that was part of it. "And," I said,
"you were nineteen."
We talked of first impressions of each other. I told
her that of all the waitresses I bussed for, she was the
only one who asked if she might stack the dishes to
make them easier for me to carry. I had made a good
impression, too, she said. So, she had been shocked to
later see the *New York Times* story saying I had been
expelled from Yale.

What she had seen was a report that six freshmen had been expelled from Yale for rioting, and somehow—I suspect it was
started by the *Yale Daily News*—were being called "the unholy
six." I wish I could say we had been demonstrating against

something like fascism, but we were just freshmen simply letting off steam before the Christmas recess. For sport, many were tossing toilet paper from their dorm windows, draping it on trees. My sin was a failed attempt to hit a streetlight with an ink bottle. Others had tried and missed, so I had tried, too.

Despite the two or three hundred freshmen participating in this foolishness, campus cops caught only six of us. A month later the entire Class of 1935 pledged never to cause such mischief again, and we "unholies" were reinstated. Still, only one besides me came back. The rest had either transferred to other universities or regarded making up a month's assignments too formidable an undertaking.

Lois said, "I couldn't believe it; I had to write to you. You
    wrote back, and that was the beginning of everything."
    She said that until then she hadn't given me a whole lot
    of thought. "Then I found myself looking forward to
    your letters."

It's curious: for most of that summer we first met, I thought of Lois simply as likable. No thought of romance entered my head. Then there was the evening in mid-August when, out of nowhere, came this road-to-Damascus thing—the moment, I swear, that Lois mesmerized me.

It was a Saturday night. Lois was cleaning off her tables and I was standing at the far end of the dining room watching. I saw her all at once as absolutely lovely, and growing in me was a great big desire to take her to the movies, to be with her. This was not like anything I had ever experienced. Greta Garbo's latest was being shown that night in Northfield's town hall. To go with Lois to see the film, to be with her, mattered so much the room filled with mist. She moved among the tables, wiping them with a damp cloth, in this mist. There was, of course, no mist, but for me it was real—is still real. As I write I can see the mist as I did then, filling the room, surrounding her. I begin to understand how people see visions.

I watched and finally summoned the courage to go to her, for she was a college woman and I a schoolboy. "Oh, I'm sorry," she said, "I have a date." Then I saw him waiting. It was Dick Williams, the good-looking junior from Amherst.

Lois and I worked together only one more week, but I would not have asked her again if we had had ten weeks. I had stepped out of bounds. Prep schoolers didn't date college sophomores.

When Christmas came I mailed a card to Lois at her home address in Wagram, North Carolina. She mailed one back, including news that her father had died in an automobile accident. (She didn't tell me that, lying alongside him at the hospital in Laurenburg, she had given two quarts of blood in an effort to save him.) We exchanged greetings the next Christmas; and it was two weeks after that Christmas—in mid-January 1932—I got her attention the hard way in the *New York Times*.

It could be we owe our marriage to Christmas and the traditional exchange of greetings. We exchanged cards for seven years until 1937, when, traveling by Greyhound bus to Miami, I stopped off in Raleigh to see her. She was teaching fourth and fifth graders at the State School for the Blind, and I saw her teaching. I saw how patiently she taught. I saw her love for the children and their love for her, how their blind faces brightened at the sound of her voice about the campus. I visited for two days. It was when I got back to the *Citizen* in Columbus that we began corresponding.

None of the letters from that time has survived, probably because nothing was expected to come of them. I do have notes, however, taken from one letter. Lois quoted three amusing mistakes her blind students had made while typing, and I had copied them and the names of the students. They are:

"We sailed northeasy."

"Let's go violence picking."

"Rome was noted for its toads."

It was like her to name the students. They were George, Anne, and Duncan in that order. I was nourished by her humor from the start.

For two years we wrote to each other every few months. We ended our letters "Sincerely" and "Your friend," but then I began feeling something beyond friendship, something close to longing. When we exchanged pictures I found myself looking often at her picture. I didn't tell her I loved her. I didn't know I loved her until later when I discovered she loved me. Then it broke upon me. Big bang.

That moment was about five-thirty in the afternoon of October 2, 1939. I had spent spring and summer in France gathering material for what I enjoyed calling the Great French Novel. It had been a pleasant time cut off by the outbreak of World War II and the expiration of my six-month leave from the Columbus paper. I knew Ralph Heinzen, chief of the United Press bureau in Paris, and probably could have gone to work for U.P., perhaps could have become a war correspondent—Heinzen was short-handed—but feeling more enthusiastic than ever about the book with my research complete, I had to come home and write it.*

---

* The title of the book was *Object of Art*. After rejection by a dozen publishers, I gave it up.

What happened that early evening in October 1939 was that I found in my mailbox a letter Lois had mailed to me care of American Express in Paris, and that American Express had forwarded. A most precious letter. It cried out her anxiety for my safety, showed nakedly her love. Through my apartment window, the sunset was splashing all over me as I whooped and hollered, leaping about the room shouting, "She loves me! She loves me! She loves me!" I was crazy with joy. I guess it was my most joyous moment.

I telephoned her. I said I was safe and loved her. She said she loved me, and I told her I couldn't come right then—I was just back at work—but I'd write every day and be down to see her no later than Christmas. I still have some of those every-day letters, hers and mine, and I tell you, we were in love.

JUNE 17: Tonight when I told Lois I loved her, she said, "Thank you." My God.

JULY 2: A letter from Cronkite saying, "Despite everything, I pray you both have room in which to enjoy life." We do find enjoyment in unexpected ways. It's perceptive of Cronkite to think we can still do that. We're experiencing something significant in life, about life, not just in our lives.

JULY 7: Lois is now in Room 208. A good thing about the room is that she can see sunsets from her bed. They show ablaze between the trees and remind her of sunsets seen through the long-leaf pine back home.

JULY 9: From the menus given Lois, I find that she's on a regular diet. Because of her confusion with multiple

choices, I discuss the offerings with her and then circle
what she wants.

JULY 16: Today for her eighty-seventh birthday, I gave
Lois a white cotton blouse—she's lovely in white—and
a poor poem.

I am grateful
Dear, sweet lady,
I had my life
With you to share
Thought of never
Having known you
I could not bear.

Two weeks later on my birthday, she gave me her poem, composed with so much effort and, I must believe, so much love.

She got the pen and paper from a nurse's aide. No poem
has meant, or ever will mean, as much to me as this one.

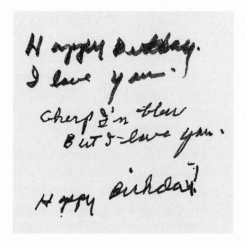

JULY 25: As I ate breakfast, I felt excited. I had a sense of happy expectation but couldn't figure why. Then I realized what it was. The sun was shining, so I could go with Lois to our bench. I would be alone with her in the woods. *I would be with her.*

AUGUST 5: I'm tired. I have been going to see Lois after breakfast, then around four in the afternoon, and again at bedtime, which is the sweetest time. For some reason, it's in the morning I most often find her crying. This is no ordinary crying, but crying so wrenching as to be scarcely bearable, so loud I hear it as I approach her room, before I open the door. Anne says I should skip these morning visits that tear me, and I'm going to. I feel I must. But, I am miserable in the decision.

AUGUST 10: Lois wants to help, to give in some way as she always has given. There was a tender moment this afternoon when she reached up from her wheelchair to straighten my tie. Oh, the wonderment of that simple gesture. If I give her a peppermint, she takes a small bite and then passes it to me. I never give her a cookie but she wants to share it. When she began doing this, I would say, "No, honey, it's for you." How blind of me! Self-centered, too. I am diabetic and my first thought had been not of Lois wanting to share, but of sugar.

SEPTEMBER 6: I fouled up. I was thinking of a piece of writing I wanted to get back to and started to leave Lois as soon as she was settled in bed. I heard a small cry and looked back. She was holding out her hand. I had forgotten for a moment that at bedtime, before she slept, we always held hands. I don't know how I could have forgotten that.

I stayed, and holding her hand, looking at her, I thought of our long time together. I thought of our loving. I thought of our dreams. I thought of the mundane: the thousands of glasses of orange juice she must have squeezed; how, before we had a washer, she must have washed diapers hundreds of times; I thought of how many ways she had used that hand I was holding. I thought of her devotion, what I owe her, what I owe God for allowing me her love.

SEPTEMBER 18: I'm so glad the nurses like Lois. It means not only better care, but a more pleasant atmosphere. A nurse told me today, "When I see your wife and ask how she's doing, she gives me this smile and a thumbs-up. Always the thumbs-up. I love it." It's not quite like that with nurse's aides. While some are caring, others perform like automatons. No smiling, no touching; just a job.

SEPTEMBER 27: Warm autumnal day, ideal for dispensing cashew nuts to the squirrels that come to our bench. Lois is impressed by how provident they are. After eating its fill, each squirrel, tail afloat, dashes off to bury for another day whatever leftover nut it can grab. Lois greatly enjoys this scene. She does have room, as Cronkite hoped, in which to enjoy life.

OCTOBER 4: A stellar day for Lois: surrounded at Sunday dinner by more family than any time in years. This is

because Rob and Diana are down from Connecticut
and were joined at the table by our grandson, Andrew,
and, of course, by Anne, Tom, and me; seven in all. We
chattered away, Lois listening, no sadness allowed.

Rob, who works in marketing, married our younger daughter,
Lois, who died young and left us the two granddaughters, Lisa
and Alison. So, Diana is Rob's second wife, successful busi-
nesswoman and caring stepmother for the two girls, who are
now in their thirties. One of the last letters my Lois wrote was
to Diana expressing appreciation and love.

OCTOBER 22: A nurse called at 2:50 P.M. to say that Lois
   had fallen again but did not seem to have hurt herself.
   I went down immediately. The nurses change shifts at
   3 P.M., and whoever had called was gone when I
   arrived. The nurse on duty had no more information. I
   don't think Lois was hurt, but she still has back pain
   from the fall several weeks ago. They're going to give
   her some kind of therapeutic treatment for that next
   week. After the fall this afternoon, we had a good time
   in the sun.

OCTOBER 26: Tonight I read to her—so many years my
   editor—a chapter I had a difficult time writing. It was a
   long chapter, but she stayed awake and then, I won't
   forget, wanted to hold it. She held it as though the
   pages were holy. I broke down.

OCTOBER 27: We had just kissed goodnight when she
   reached up and held my face in both hands. Her hands

were gentle as an angel's, and she held my face for a long time.

OCTOBER 28: Lois's wedding ring has disappeared. Everyone is looking for it.

OCTOBER 29: The ring is still missing. I have drawn a sketch of the ring and posted it at the nurses' station.

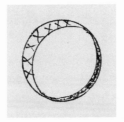

Lost: Wedding Ring.
Slipped from Lois Bliss's finger sometime early on
Wednesday, October 28, 1998.
Platinum. Set with seven small diamonds.

I had paid $85 for the ring. It was displayed in the middle of the jeweler's window in Columbus and I knew the instant I saw it that it was the ring for Lois, so looked at no others. Four years before her death, when she was still getting about, she took the ring to a jeweler to see whether any of the seven little diamonds were damaged. She wanted it right for Anne. Two were found to be cracked, and replacing them cost twice the amount the ring had cost in 1940. Still, that $85 in 1940 was two weeks' pay at the paper.

OCTOBER 30: Tonight when I stopped reading McNeill's poems, Lois ever so softly recited a verse she says appears on his tombstone, the same verse we often recited together when we prayed at night:

O Lord, we know so little what is best;
Wingless we move so lowly.
But in Thy all-knowledge let us rest,
O, holy, holy, holy.

Lois's parents lie in the same cemetery as John Charles McNeill.

OCTOBER 31: Lois has her wedding ring. An aide brought it to me, saying she had found it under the bed and taken it home, but felt so uncomfortable she had to bring it back. What surprises me is how frank she was. I told her that what she had done in bringing it back was rather wonderful.

NOVEMBER 1: A good time today with Anne and Tom, who came over after church. Instead of going downstairs, I fixed one of my stir-fry dinners, making a cozy family affair. Lois enjoyed every minute.

NOVEMBER 2: She fell again tonight. Escaped with a bruised elbow, but it couldn't have helped her back. The nurses say she fell while undressing herself for bed. An aide is supposed to do that, but Lois may have grown impatient.

NOVEMBER 3: As Lois was eating, she suddenly said, "I
   want to kiss you." Does make a fellow feel good.

NOVEMBER 4: Yesterday I voted alone in an election for
   the first time since we married. No political arguments
   at our house. We are Democrats to the core.

We did argue, of course, and she could get pretty mad at me.
I've been trying to remember the times she did get vexed,
and I'm surprised by what comes to mind first. We were sail-
ing tourist (more like steerage) on a crock of a ship called the
Vulcania. It was stormy, typical of the Atlantic in early spring—
so stormy that looking out our porthole, half the time we had
an underwater view.

The porthole leaked. Not a deluge, but enough so that
waking one morning, we could hear a slight sloshing when
the ship rolled. What aroused Lois's ire—real ire—was
when, on the first morning out of New York, I found water
on the floor and squandered Lois's precious facial tissues
soaking it up.

I do have a dickens of a time recalling when we fussed.
They were two-bit fusses, easy to forget.

NOVEMBER 6: She wouldn't go to sleep. I read poetry,
   must have sung "In the Garden" four or five times, said
   goodnight I don't know how many times, and after
   more than an hour gave up. I was going out the door
   when she called to me. I was tired. And annoyed.
   "What *is* it?" I said. "I love you," she said. You'd think
   by now I would have learned patience.

NOVEMBER 26: Thanksgiving Day. Lois, in her best
dress, joined Anne, Tom, Andrew and his girl friend
Susan,* and me, for dinner in the residents' dining
room, an occasion we all enjoyed. Lois needs help in
eating. I fed her—sparingly, I fear, not wishing to
embarrass her.

NOVEMBER 28: My Lois has not lost her sense of humor.
This afternoon she made a very long speech, of which I
understood not a word. "Will you swear to that?" I
asked, and she laughed. So, there I have another reason
for loving this woman: she can laugh at herself.

NOVEMBER 30: All day we felt close, but tonight
especially. A wind had come up, and we sat by the
window watching the silhouettes of trees swaying, an
arboreal ballet, the tops of them dancing.
   "Beautiful," I whispered.
   A long silence, and then, taking my hand, she said,
"You and me."

The Reverend Barbara Gerlach of the First Congregational
United Church of Christ in Washington, learning of Lois's re-
mark, used it in a sermon. She said, "God is telling us to turn
to the person on our right and on our left and across the street
and across the world, and say to each of them, 'You and me,
you and me, you and me. . .'" In her illness, Lois still managed
to give hope to others.

* Susan and Andrew were married in June 2001.

DECEMBER 1: I find that Lois is wearing someone else's
glasses. These are rimless. I've asked everyone on the
floor to please watch out for her pair. Two days ago
one of her slippers also disappeared. Still no sign of it.

DECEMBER 3: Lois has her glasses back. They were found
in another patient's room. I guess it's goodbye to the
slipper.

After Lois died, I dreaded looking into her closets: all those
dresses, coats, jackets, shoes, all the memories associated with
what she wore. Getting rid of them seemed beyond what I
could do, and then, all of a sudden, there stood Anne at the
bedroom door with five great plastic bags, appropriately
black. She had made an appointment with the Salvation Army
and had come to gather up the clothes. I was spared that.

The clothes were soon gone, but earrings, necklaces, lock-
ets, brooches, bracelets, handkerchiefs, scarves, purses, and
medicines remained. In disposing of possessions such as these,
nothing inflicted as much pain as the disposal of Lois's glasses.
I took them to a cardboard box in the lobby, close by the front
desk. The box has a slit in the top and a sign that reads: "The
glasses you don't need may help someone to see." My teacher
of blind children would want that. But to take the glasses she
wore until the day of her death, something so intimate as to be
almost a part of her, and to part with them was terribly hard.
With a "bless you," I put them in the box. I heard them drop
and got away as quickly as I could.

DECEMBER 6: I'm surprised to find that one of the best
times is when I come down and find Lois asleep. I sit

and watch, and quite often she wakes and smiles. She smiles so lovingly I'm reminded of the old song, "I'd Walk a Mile for One of Your Smiles." There are these wonderful moments.

DECEMBER 8: Temperatures this December day rose into the high seventies. Lois and I got out into the garden, probably for the last time this season; the high tomorrow is supposed to be in the mid-fifties.

DECEMBER 9: Before going down to get the mail I asked Lois if she had to go to the bathroom. Each time I asked she made a speech, none of which was understandable. I begged her, "Just say yes or no. Making speeches will get you nowhere." She laughed at that, and then wouldn't say anything. I put her on the john anyway and am damn glad I did.

DECEMBER 13: Attended Sunday service with Lois, something I rarely do because I'm trying very hard to finish rewriting *Physician for Shaowu*.* This special service for patients is held in the infirmary and consists mostly of hymn-singing. The hymns are printed on sheets of paper so patients can hold them more easily, and it is touching to see how patients suffering from dementia, and who cannot read, strive to sing along with those who can. Today we sang two

---

* The biography of my father, published by John Wiley & Sons in 2001 with the title *Beyond the Stone Arches*.

of Lois's favorites, "In the Garden" and "Amazing Grace." She took my hand at the start of the service and held it to the end. I will come to these services more often.

DECEMBER 19: Anne brought take-out Chinese, and we had supper listening to talk about impeaching the president. I sang to Lois when she had gone to bed. Again it was her favorite hymn, Miles's "In the Garden." All day I was unable to understand anything she said, but after I sang, she said softly, almost perfectly, "You have a lovely voice." It was the first time she ever said that—and it was news to me. God, I love her.

DECEMBER 21: 1:35 P.M. Just came up from putting Lois down for a nap. As I tucked her in I said, "You know, you're a beautiful person." And she said slowly, "So . . . I . . . have . . . been . . . told."

Tonight I took her to the main dining room for a candlelight dinner. She was greeted there by many friends.

This was Lois's last meal in the main dining room. I often pass by the table where we sat and picture how it was.

DECEMBER 25: Again we spent most of Christmas at Anne and Tom's. Instead of a star on top of the Christmas tree, Anne had the little angel we put at the top of our trees when she was a girl. I saw Lois looking at it. I know she remembered.

DECEMBER 26: Lois's wheelchair, No. 52, keeps disappearing from her room. This afternoon nurse's aides and I spent twenty minutes looking for it, and these are precious minutes: because Lois takes a nap, and then supper is served at five o'clock, I have only an hour or so to be with her in the afternoon.

DECEMBER 27: Bedtime is still the most precious time, although about the only way we can express how we feel is by holding hands. She holds my hand as often as I hold hers. I feel at home in her hand.

DECEMBER 29: Lois's wheelchair was missing again yesterday, so I have made a sign, ten inches by fourteen inches, and fastened it with surgical tape to the back of her chair: "This chair assigned to Lois Bliss."

DECEMBER 30: Well, I've been spanked. An officious staff person caught Lois and me in the auditorium this afternoon and suggested I remove the sign, saying, "Surely, Mr. Bliss, you know better than that."

I kept the sign but made it smaller, and the chair stopped disappearing.

DECEMBER 31: I kept my sweetheart up late so we could see the old year out. We watched as the crowd in Times Square chanted and the glittering ball gradually came down. My old CBS colleague Bob Trout, speaking from an Astor Hotel balcony, had been first to report this year-end ritual on television. He did it for

years. Trout hated the cold out there on the balcony—
the cold anywhere—and retired to balmy Spain. As we
watched, Lois said, "I miss Bob Trout." I do, too.

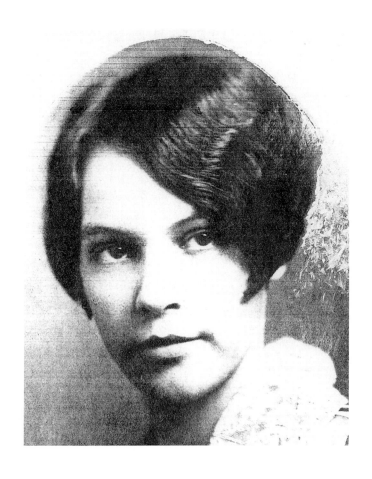

Lois Arnette, Meredith College, Raleigh, North Carolina, 1928.

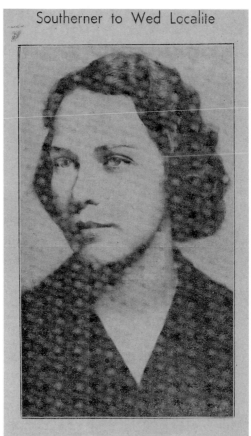

MRS. JOHN MADISON ARNETTE of Raleigh, N. C., announces the engagement of her daughter, Lois, to Edward L. Bliss Jr. of Columbus, son of Dr. and Mrs. Edward L. Bliss of Oberlin, O. The bride-elect is a graduate of Mere- dith College and is at present a teacher in the North Carolina State School for the Blind. Mr. Bliss attended preparatory school at Mount Hermon, Mass., and was gradu- ated from Yale University. He is now a member of the editorial staff of The Citizen.

Our wedding announcement in *The Columbus Citizen*, July 1940.

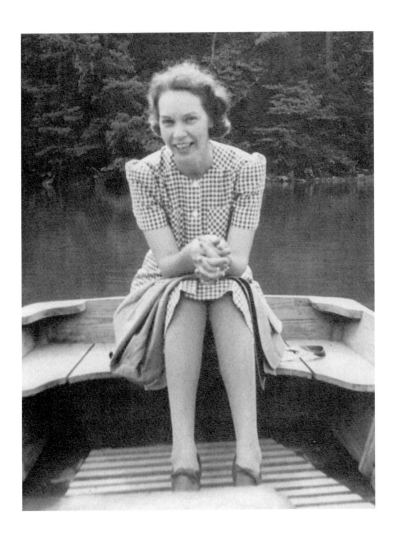

Lois Arnette Bliss at Lake Lure, North Carolina, August 27, 1940,
the day after our wedding.

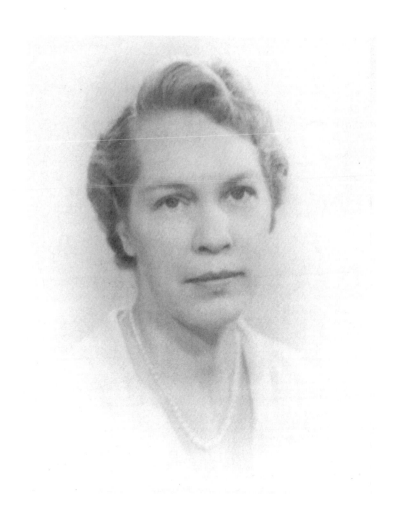

Lois, circa 1963.

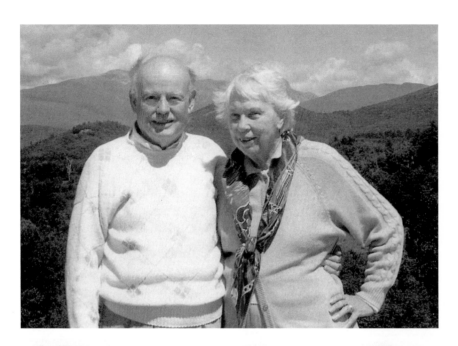

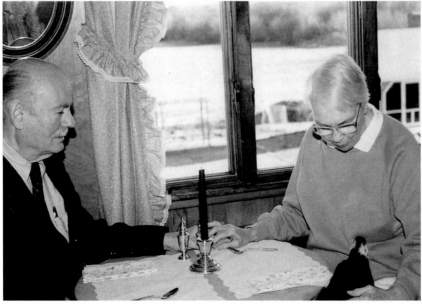

Above: Vacationing in North Conway, New Hampshire, 1984.
Below: Dinner out and a dog.

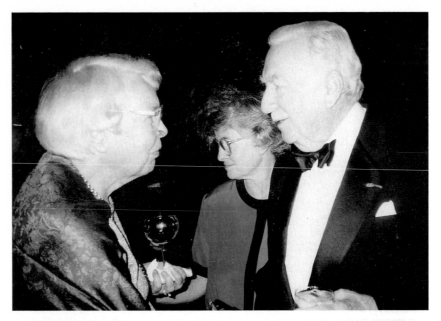

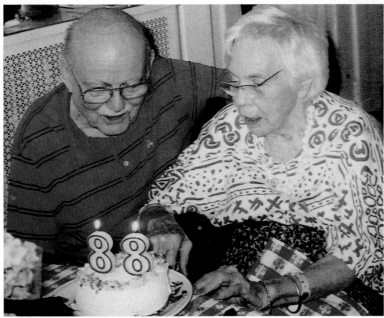

Above: Lois with Walter Cronkite, friend Louisa Stone in center, Miami Beach, 1993.
Below: Eighty-eighth birthday at Anne's, July 16, 1999.

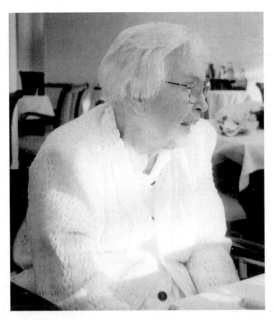

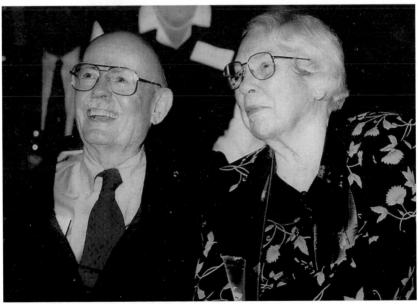

Above: Lois enjoying dinner in the main dining room at the Goodwin House.
We did not know it was for the last time.
Below: Our last night out together, American University, May 9, 1996.

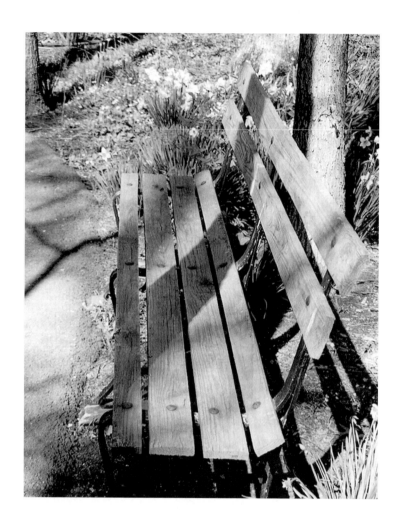

Our place in the woods.

1999

After fifty-eight years, this was our last whole year. It's good we didn't know; the knowledge would have hovered over us, adding poignancy to the already poignant. So, not knowing, yet knowing, we went on day by day, doing mostly what we had been doing.

Lois was weaker now, but she still fed herself, washed her own hands, brushed her own teeth. But she spoke less. One day, with great difficulty, she repeated one of her favorite stories. It was about how, back in the 1930s, there was a woman—an English professor at Elon College—who volunteered to lead cheers for the football team. "One day she got up in front of the stands and said, 'All right now. Not too loud, just loud enough to be heard. Rah! Rah! Rah!'" Lois loved that "not too loud." She still enjoyed a good story.

Lois and I still had some wonderful, happy moments. We had kissing places. One was just inside the Alzheimer's unit. A large picture of a tree hangs on the wall there. When we came to this picture I would say, "Now under the boughs of the Kissin' Tree, we gotta kiss." She would laugh and I would get a good kiss. The other place was a few feet down the hall from our apartment. If no one was around, I'd stop the wheelchair and kiss her. It thrilled me when she kissed me back. She could still do that to me.

My first entry for 1999 was about this kissing.

JANUARY 3: We kiss a lot. Sometimes she kisses most solemnly as though for the last time. Yesterday she kissed as though the kisses were a kind of affirmation: that she is still herself, and we *are* together. I know today we kissed for the pleasure of it.

JANUARY 4: It's not always sweetness. Tonight, after a good time together, I told Lois I had to leave, and she said angrily, "All right, leave!" Of course, I stayed.

I recall only one other scene like that.

JANUARY 6: No more Lois watching over me. Last night in the middle of the night, I got cold and put on an extra blanket. I think of how, during similar cold nights in the past, I would wake to feel the blue lightweight blanket she bought when we were first married being laid over the length of me.

JANUARY 7: Lois had a mammogram taken today at
Alexandria Hospital. This was done, I suppose, because
of her breast cancer in 1986. But, goodness, she has
Alzheimer's. My darling is dying.

Lois had lost her right breast to cancer. She had a fine surgeon.
He had called on her the morning following the operation
and, after examining her, went to a straight chair by the window,
sat down, and started to cry. None of us spoke. After about a
minute he got up and left. Not long after that he gave up
surgery to teach at the Boston University School of Medicine.
Lois had lovely breasts. I have wondered whether, psychologi-
cally, his disfigurement of women had become more than he
could bear.

JANUARY 8: One of the women in the infirmary beauty
shop fixes Lois's hair beautifully. She's awfully nice. I
wish Lois had her every time.

JANUARY 9: I have added "Blue Skies" to my repertoire
at bedtime. I learned it as a teenager. The other songs
I attempt, along with "In the Garden," are "There's a
Long, Long Trail Awinding" and "Roses Are
Blooming in Piccardy." The nights I don't sing, she
goes to sleep listening to a Tchaikovsky recording. All
kinds of good stuff on it, such as "Andante Cantabile"
and "Chanson Triste."

JANUARY 10: It's getting hard, here in the apartment,
seeing all around me the things Lois used and won't

use again: the chair where she sat, the bed where she slept, the comb and brush on the bureau, the earrings. I find myself disposing of things she'll never need, such as old bras and almost-empty tubes of hand lotion. Ridiculous how this hurts.

JANUARY 13: Lois received a letter today saying, "The results of your recent diagnostic mammogram indicate no suspicion of breast cancer." The letter—it has to be a form letter—recommends that she continue with annual examinations. More absurdity. More waste of Medicare money.

JANUARY 28: Lois is now in Room 214 on the second floor. Like our apartment on the fifth floor, it's next to the stairwell, so I often skip the elevator and walk down. Her roommate has a private nurse, a lovely woman from Ecuador. Like so many people, she's picked up the habit of sprinkling her sentences with "you knows." She is so kind—twice I've found her polishing Lois's nails. This old fellow gave her a free lecture, and I do believe she is cured; I haven't heard a "you know" from her for a long time. She is serious about learning.

Lois's roommate is Jacqueline Turner. They say she has many friends, but I've seen no visitors. When she's not sitting she lies, a bundle, in fetal position on her bed. She is helpless.

There are residents, good friends of patients, who can't bring themselves to come to the second floor because that is probably where they will die. I am surprised by friends who apologize for not coming to visit Lois by saying, "I just can't stand it there."

FEBRUARY 7: Kind note from Andy Rooney saying he had tried unsuccessfully to find my phone number. He said that although he never has been close to anyone with Alzheimer's, he understands how terrible it is. He also offered anecdotal stuff for a book I want to write about the glory days of CBS News. He and I are among the few left who were there.

FEBRUARY 15: Yesterday Lois fell and suffered a good gash in her forehead. It happened in a second-floor lounge where, along with four or five other patients, she was watching television. No nurse or nurse's aide was present, so when she had to go to a bathroom, she struck out for what she thought was one across the hall. It was in trying to get through the door that she fell.

I was called and found Lois, face streaked with blood, in her wheelchair. A nurse was applying an ice pack to the cut. I demanded to know what had happened. Two aides said they didn't see her because they were caring for other patients. "We're short-handed," they said. Another interjected that she was working in the food area, so couldn't see what was going on. At this point, Lois began vomiting. Then she began bleeding from the nose. I expressed my anxiety and was told an ambulance was on the way. At Alexandria Hospital, a CAT scan showed no concussion. A doctor closed the cut with seven stitches, and an ambulance brought Lois back to Goodwin House around midnight.

Today, with some anger, I sent the director of nursing a memorandum. I said in my last paragraph: "I make this report cognizant of, and grateful for, the caring people who work on the second floor. And, as they say, what's done is done, but obviously where there is a group of patients, someone should be watching. What happened last night comes close to neglect." In reply I received an expression of regret over the accident, and assurance that corrective steps have been taken.

FEBRUARY 18: Kathy Durham, a Goodwin House social worker, came to talk to me. She wondered how I was coping. About all I could say was that although, of course, I hurt, I believed I was "handling it." I told her Lois's courage helped, that she inspired me, and that I was praying a lot. She said she would stay in touch.

MARCH 14: I especially enjoyed supper with Lois. She seemed happy and practically gulped down my stir-fry. We watched *60 Minutes* and, as always, learned from Mike Wallace. I remember he hugged Lois when he saw her at the RTNDA convention in 1991, the year he received the Paul White Award.

MARCH 18: Took Lois to the ninth-floor sun parlor where, through the floor-to-ceiling windows, we have a grand panoramic view of Washington: the National

Cathedral on the far left, the dome of the Capitol on the right, and the Washington Monument in between. Because spring is almost here, we saw all shades of green, a verdant spectrum stretching from our woods to the distant hills of Maryland. I don't know why we don't go up to that sun parlor more often. Such a view, and it's free.

MARCH 27: Alison, Wayne, and great-granddaughter, Alexandra, here for dinner. Often when they come down from Connecticut, they visit one of Alison's college friends who lives near here. When I asked Alison if they were going on to see her, she said, "This time, we came just to see Lady. We'll be over again tomorrow." I feel so grateful to Alison for that.

APRIL 22: Marauders have desecrated our bench, scribbling all over it with spray paint. Most words are indecipherable, none obscene. *Pimp* is the naughtiest word.

MAY 12: Today Lois moved from the infirmary to the new ward for Alzheimer's patients on the first floor. She has a private room—one we chose weeks ago—which has two large windows looking out into the woods. She knew the transfer was coming and was glad for it. I feel good that Lois has this.

This special unit—I hate its name, Hope Garden—proved a pleasant place with period furniture, marvelous paintings, and a private courtyard with flowering shrubs. Rooms for

Alzheimer's patients line this comfortable space. And the unit has pets. Besides a couple of parakeets that mate regularly, producing baby parakeets, it has a tomcat, Caper, and a very lazy, very sweet Labrador retriever named Penny. Caper, with an air of importance, patrols the ward, thinks he's boss. How Lois would have loved for him to jump into her lap and nestle there, but that's beneath him. Penny, on the other hand, loves everybody.

MAY 15: Today I bought two large posters to hang in
      Lois's new room. One is a watercolor of Bar Harbor
      with colorful, mostly pink flowers in the foreground,
      then blue water, and a spit of land beyond. The other
      picture, more somber, looks like a Colorado scene,
      with a swift-running brook and a high mountain. In the
      sky are three billowy clouds.
            I said to Lois, "Those are smoke signals. Do you
      know what they're saying?"
            "No."
            "They're saying, 'I love you.'"
            I hung them on the walls; the harbor scene at the
      head of Lois's bed and the poster with smoke signals on
      the wall facing her.

After Lois's death I took the "smoke signal" poster down to our art center, thinking that residents taking painting lessons might like to copy it. I was touched a week later when I found it had been framed and hung in one of the center's offices.

MAY 18: I'm impressed by the array of activities in the
      Alzheimer's unit. After morning exercises (conducted

sitting down) there may be art class, a history quiz,
putting for golfers, or baking. When I went to see Lois
this morning she and another woman were stirring
milk into some kind of cake mix.

A favorite afternoon game is bingo, and I am struck
by how beautifully Michelle, the therapist, makes a
patient's mistake with numbers seem like no mistake at
all. Volunteers also often come to entertain in the
afternoon. In just the short time Lois has been there
she has heard a barbershop quartet and a guitarist who
sang old hymns. When there isn't this entertainment,
the television set is on. Here, too, the old Shirley
Temple movies and Lawrence Welk's music are played
from videotapes. Each day the unit's schedule also
includes "cocktails" at four o'clock. The word is
misleading: any patient asking for a martini will get
apple juice or a Coke.

Observing other Alzheimer's patients, I learned how greatly
their symptoms vary. Some patients rarely spoke; others
were loquacious. Some sat; others paced the ward, remind-
ing me of caged animals. And although a few—very few—
chafed at restrictions—"Why can't I go out that door?"—
other patients accepted them readily. Some had no idea they
were ill. One patient, a woman of about eighty, asked me
how long I had worked "in this factory." I said, "Eleven
years," the length of time I had resided at Goodwin House,
and she said brightly, "Well, it's a good place to work." I
watched her walk away. She walked with no difficulty, and
I had an ugly thought: how come she can walk like that and
Lois can't?

But Lois had understanding. She knew where she was, who she was, and who I was. Even when she lost her ability to speak, communication by gesture—caress, hand clasp, kiss—served better than I ever had imagined possible.

JUNE 1: I don't understand. She's sophisticated, but no matter how bad the joke is, she laughs. The latest: Why does the man in the picture look so upset? They framed him, then had him hung.

JUNE 6: This afternoon as I was taking Lois to the mailroom, a waitress coming on duty stopped and kissed her. This is a beautiful young Ethiopian woman, an immigrant who waited on us when Lois was well. Often we meet fellow residents who stop briefly and either ask Lois how she is, or tell her how well she looks—"How *pretty* you are today!" One woman, meaning well, talks baby talk. I say nothing, but, God, I cringe.

By now we had fallen into a routine so that each day around four o'clock, I took Lois to get the mail. I would give her letters and magazines to hold in her lap and then, if the weather allowed it, wheel her up the garden path to the woods where, sitting together, she in her wheelchair and me on the bench, I read her the mail. She particularly enjoyed hearing from her sister Jo, who wrote once a week on notepaper featuring the great French painters like Renoir and Monet. Squirrels visited us, and I kept wishing I had brought peanuts. (I did once.) If the weather was bad, we sat in the Goodwin House parlor, almost always by ourselves.

After reading the mail and enjoying some precious time just being together, we usually went up to our apartment, caught the *Headline News* at four-thirty, and watched the last half of *Murder She Wrote*. I took her down to the infirmary dining room a little after five. Then we were together again at bedtime.

JUNE 20: I don't go out to movies anymore—it would be no fun without her. The last movie we saw together was *Fly Away Home*, the lovely story of a girl who rescues Canada goose eggs from a bulldozer. She raises the hatched goslings, of course. Using his airplane, the girl's father teaches the young geese to fly, and when it's time to migrate they fly away with the father escorting them. If we had planned a last movie, we couldn't have done better.

JUNE 26: Lois has lost more than thirty pounds. When I lay down with her tonight, I felt her wrist. It was like sticks wrapped in skin.

JUNE 28: We are enjoying each other, no matter what. We have our bench. We waste not the kissin' places, and we have our jokes. We're sweethearts.

JULY 2: Naz, the RN from Iran, said today that she is impressed by my devotion. I'm grateful to her for that. I visit Lois only twice a day and, because I am so near, I do feel guilty for not doing so more often.

JULY 15: A dentist has started coming to Goodwin House, and today Lois had her teeth cleaned. No cavities.

JULY 16: Lois's eighty-eighth birthday, and another good time at Anne and Tom's. Andrew is home from the University of Georgia with a brand-new MBA, and I could tell Lois is proud of him.

Anne took pictures. In one, Lois is laughing after blowing out the candles. Other photos show her opening Anne's present: a light, loose-knit blanket, perfect for afternoon naps. But one picture of her looking at the blanket troubles me. She showed a happy face when she first saw the blanket, but in this picture taken moments later, she appears terribly solemn. It's not a look of disappointment, but of sadness. I wonder what she was thinking.

AUGUST 2: She gave me a kiss, a very wet one, and when she couldn't see me behind her wheelchair, I wiped it off. I'm sorry I did that.

AUGUST 8: Tonight at bedtime, Lois moved her lips in prayer. It is such a special thing, because for weeks she has just listened.

AUGUST 16: I have bought a radio for her, a small one she can tuck under her pillow and listen to at night. I set it for a public station so that all my weakened news buff has to do to hear *Morning Edition* or *All Things Considered* is turn it on.

AUGUST 26: An aide found Lois breathing in gasps. She was given oxygen, and her breathing returned to normal.

This was our fifty-ninth wedding anniversary, but strangely I find no reference to this in my notes, nor do I have any recollection of it. We celebrated, I fear, hardly at all. And it was our last.

OCTOBER 15: I've seen again and again how a joke can change Lois's disposition. *She loves jokes.* Because she looked downhearted this afternoon, I told her the experience of the Yankee traveling man one hot night in Atlanta. It was before air conditioning, and the Yankee, after showering and putting on a clean shirt, went down to the hotel dining room for dinner.

"Could you bring me a nice cold martini?" he asked.

"Yes, sir," the waiter said. "Would you like a regular martini or a martini special?"

"What's the difference?"

"Well, sir, with a martini special you get grits."

Lois laughed. Wonderful laugh. The nurse Naz, fixing Lois after her nap, didn't laugh, but turned to me: "You see, Mrs. Bliss understands everything. I don't think she has Alzheimer's."

Well, John Bayley's Iris had Alzheimer's, and he says she "feasted" on every bit of information he gave her. I think with this disease, as with most, it's hard to draw a line. I think, too, how awareness of her condition must be difficult for Lois, but she, like Iris, does not complain. Bayley says Iris didn't seem to know *how* to complain. I doubt that with Lois. She had no trouble letting us know her back hurt after a fall in the bathroom. But never in conversation has she in any way bemoaned her fate.

And that baffles me. When she could no longer read, she never said she missed reading. A year later when she could no longer write, she never said she wished she could write; and when she could no longer walk, she never said she wished she could. When she was losing her power of speech, she never spoke of losing it. She does cry, but I cannot believe this is from being sorry for herself, or she would have shown it in conversation.

OCTOBER 21: I said tonight, after she had been put to bed, "Just think, we've been married fifty-nine years." I thought she might smile or perhaps reach out her hand. Instead she looked at me most seriously, as though recalling the strivings of those years as well as the joys. I asked if she remembered the day I proposed and the trouble we had. Now she smiled.

It was December 17, 1939, and again I had driven down to Raleigh. That morning walking in Hillsborough Street to the State School for the Blind, I went into—somehow was drawn into—a church. And there, sitting in a back pew, I asked God's help because it was such a big thing I was about to do. I don't know what I said that morning in the church, but late that afternoon, toward evening, parked by the side of State Route 40, Lois said she would marry me.

Proposal in such a spot hadn't been my plan. Earlier that afternoon I had driven with Lois into a park and was about to propose when an officer came over and bellowed, "Break it up! The park's closed." We left. Neither of us spoke. As I drove I kept looking for a wooded area, a proper place to turn in to. I didn't find one. So, I proposed beside the state highway, practically in the weeds, because I could wait no longer.

There is another story from that time. It was while driving to Raleigh to propose that I met the man I'll always think of as Santa Claus. High in the West Virginia mountains, a few miles beyond Beckley, I came upon him hitchhiking. He wasn't wearing a red suit, but he had a plump figure and, getting in the car, he gave a laugh that, stretching only slightly, you could call merry. When I asked how far he was going, he said, "Raleigh," and I told him, "Well, you've got a ride all the way."

The man appeared somewhere in his sixties and was trying to find work in Raleigh where, he said, he had connections. He asked why I was going to Raleigh, and I told him. We became friends as we rode. When he said he had no place to stay that night, I invited him to share my room at the bed-and-breakfast where I had a reservation, and he accepted.

The next morning when I looked over to his bed, it was empty. Santa Claus was gone, but he had left a note on the washstand in the bathroom: "I hope you have a long, happy life together." It was unsigned.

NOVEMBER 2: Lois took a nap with me today. Getting her out of the wheelchair and onto the bed, and then shifting her to the middle of the bed, was a job. But, oh, her face after she went to sleep! Such a look of contentment, of consummate peace. I can't think of anything more sublime I've ever seen. She had not thought, ever, to be back in her own bed.

NOVEMBER 4: No "goodnight" from my lady tonight, for the first time I can remember. It hurt. Pretended I didn't notice.

NOVEMBER 8: Lois is a honey. When I went to bring her to the apartment, I found her in her wheelchair near the nurse's station. She gestured toward the nurse's station. I took her to it, and when she got the nurse's attention, she said in her dear, demolished voice, "Thank you." I looked puzzled, so the nurse explained. She had just given Lois some apple juice. I thought to myself, "What a lady!"

NOVEMBER 11: This was a rare warm day for mid-November, and we were able to go out into the sunshine. For some reason, truckers have dumped a load of gravel across the walk leading up to our woods, so I detoured, pushing Lois across the uneven turf, which wasn't easy. As we sat looking down over the garden, I told her, "Sometimes your old husband does something right." "Sometimes," she said, and laughed.

NOVEMBER 12: When I went down to see Lois this morning, she was crying uncontrollably. The psychiatrist said she did not know what else she can do and suggested the cause is organic, which is what the nurses have been saying all along. When Lois cries, other patients look at me as though I were a really mean person.

NOVEMBER 15: We made another try at taking naps together. It failed. The springs on the edge of the bed gave way with her weight, so that each time I tried, she almost slipped off. I had to give up. We both cried. It had meant so much.

I think now how I could have called an aide to help. But I didn't because it was our problem. It was private.

DECEMBER 9: Anne and I attended a meeting of the interdisciplinary team composed of the nurse, therapist, dietitian, and social worker most involved with Lois's care. We learned today that, because of Lois's loss of weight, she is being given the food supplement ReSource twice a day, and that for her frequent crying she is now taking the drug Celexa in addition to Zoloft. So that Lois will have more of what they call "muscle action," they have entered her in a small dance class! She is also being made to walk, with her walker, to and from meals. They reported that, as part of therapy, "we are allowing her to pet one of the guinea pigs, which she enjoys doing." I didn't know they have guinea pigs.

These briefings with family members are held regularly every few months, and last about fifteen minutes. Their purpose, as stated by Goodwin House, is "to review each patient's status and develop approaches that will maintain or improve the patient's function."

DECEMBER 13: Goodwin House provided transportation for Lois to see a gynecologist about a suspected uterine infection.

The Pap test proved negative. This was Lois's last trip to see a doctor. Many things were happening for the last time.

DECEMBER 14: I am surprised by how few clear pictures of Lois I have in my head. When I'm not with her and I try to remember how she looked on a particular occasion, I see her only vaguely. You would think I'd have a clear picture of her at our wedding, but I don't. This afternoon she was in the apartment, in her wheelchair, watching *Murder She Wrote*. I decided to fasten the picture of her in my mind so I would always have it. I stood away from her, registering the white hair, the bowed shoulders, the gray-blue eyes, the glasses on her nose. Now as I write I can see the hair, the shoulder, the eyes, but not the face, the sum of its parts. I don't understand that.

Still, some mental pictures are clear: the happy, confident look on her face as we drove off after our wedding, a most gratifying look for a groom to see; and the most beautiful, serene look last month as she stole that nap on her own bed. When I take naps now I often look across to that bed and, in my imagination, see her there with that indescribable expression of peace on her face. I know that when she is gone, I shall still see it. I know I shall see it and treasure it.

I now have other pictures of Lois in my head, reinforced by photographs ranging from the snapshot taken of her smiling at me from the stern of a rowboat, to one taken of us standing on the bow of the *Ile de France*. And, yes, the picture Anne took of us on Mother's Day 2000, the last picture.

DECEMBER 15: Tonight relatives joined patients in the Alzheimer's ward for the first annual Hope Garden holiday dinner, with music and song by a talented young guitarist, Bill Parsons. Lois celebrated with seconds of chocolate ice cream.

DECEMBER 16: Lois was able to attend the annual yule log ceremony in the Goodwin House parlor. Residents singing carols move in procession past the fireplace and toss a twig of holly into the fire, ridding themselves of the old year's woes. When I wheeled Lois past the fire, I was afraid she might fumble. But my sweetheart, the basketball player I married, made a perfect toss.

DECEMBER 17: We became engaged sixty years ago today. I went to Lois in the morning—couldn't wait till afternoon—and gave a little speech that made her open her arms to me and cry. Very different from our fiftieth wedding anniversary, which we spent in the bridal suite at the Willard.

DECEMBER 25: A lovely Christmas at Anne and Tom's. For Lois, I had a large framed picture of our Newburyport home. She had said it would be nice to have such a picture in her room. No material gift from her this time, but she gives me presents every day, such as the teenage smiles after we kiss.

That Christmas Lois received so many cards that I stopped pinning them up after the first twenty or so, except for one from our friend Mervin Block, a former writer for Cronkite. I taped his greeting, each letter an inch tall, on the wall close to the Colorado "smoke signals" where Lois could see it from her bed. It was like Mervin to send greetings like no other. He had come to see Lois, and she had called out, "Merv!" as she saw him come through the door. That was the first time I had heard her speak in two days. It surprised and delighted Merv that she recognized him.

**Hello, Lois.
Greetings--in
perpetuity!**
Merv

I summed up the year in my Christmas letter: "My dear Lois is dying—slowly, bravely—and we are having moments more precious than any other we have known. She cannot read, write, or walk, can barely speak, but she comprehends and is more endearing than I deserve. I see her in the infirmary briefly at night, but we spend real time together in the afternoon. During good weather in summer, we get out into the garden. Now when it's not too cold, we go to the roof garden where there's a grand view of the Capitol and the hills of Maryland beyond. But, believe me, Alzheimer's is cruel."

DECEMBER 26: An image persists. It is of Lois as I saw her last night when we were driving home from Anne's. She sat crumpled in her seat, all wilted. I think how straight she sat the day we drove off for our honeymoon, confident of the future. Now she sat as someone done in, near death.

DECEMBER 31: Every New Year's Eve since buying our first television, we have watched the ball descending the old Times Tower. It was different this time. After fixing a candlelight supper for us in the apartment—supermarket candles everywhere—I noticed Lois looking weary and took her down to bed. So, we saw the old year out in her room, watching the second hand of the clock on the wall.

2000

We were entering not only a new century, but a new millennium. On television, 100 million Americans watched it happen, this thing that would not happen again for 1,000 years. They watched, spellbound, as time zone by time zone, continent by continent, around the globe the new millennium was born.

This special century began with Lois and me together in the Alzheimer's ward, and the greatest piece of dialogue there ever was:

He: I love you.

She: I love you, too.

The first entry for the year 2000 concerns Lois's last attempt to write.

JANUARY 6: When I went to see Lois this afternoon I
found her and two other patients taking a writing test;

each had been given a marker pen and a large piece of paper, and told to write the names of people they knew. It was heartbreaking to see Lois's effort. I had told her that morning that it was the birthday of our friend Joe Allen, and it was his name, fairly recognizable, she attempted first. I can't make out the next two names, but then, quite clearly, comes my name with one *s*, and looking at it, I am deeply moved. I feel so complimented. Then she tried two more names. I think the first is that of her sister Josephine, and the second her own name. I heard Michelle say, "Mrs. Bliss, you did very well." I like Michelle. She has a nice natural way of making patients feel good about themselves.

My Lois, who had taught blind children to write with combinations of raised dots, could, herself, no longer write effectively with a pen or pencil. I still have her scribbles from that day and wish—almost wish—I didn't. But no matter what the sight of them does to me, there is no way imaginable I could bring myself to discard them.

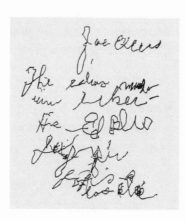

2000

JANUARY 7: Today Lucy Roberts, a patient in Lois's ward, came over to me and said, in an angel's voice, "You have a sweet wife." Well, I love Lucy Roberts. Nurses say that, like me, she was born in China and that her father, like my father, was a medical missionary and established a hospital.

JANUARY 8: Another compliment for Lois. A resident, whom I can't remember ever having seen before, stopped me and said, "Your wife is so obviously a dear person." She must have observed Lois on our trips to get the mail.

JANUARY 20: Now we have something to celebrate. John Wiley & Sons is going to publish Father's biography. The news came in a telephone call from one of their senior editors, and I ran downstairs to tell Lois, who burst into tears. She is a big part of this book. As I wrote, she edited—so well.

A year later when the first copy came, Lois was gone. I took it to the large, framed picture of her on the wall in the living room and said, "See, honey, it's here."

JANUARY 21: Just a month ago when we said our goodnight prayer, sometimes I could hear her. Now I see her lips barely moving. As recently as a week ago she was saying, "I love you, too," but now when I tell her I love her, she doesn't try to speak, but squeezes my hand.

FEBRUARY 1: I'm grateful that she has kept her sense of humor. This afternoon I was pushing her in the wheelchair and, on impulse, put on an act. Stopping, I said, "You know what I'm going to do? I'm going to walk all the way around to the front of this chair, come up in front, and kiss you." Before I could kiss her, she was laughing.

FEBRUARY 3: Today, for the first time in weeks, she tried awfully hard to tell me something, something she must believe is important for me to know. But the effort failed. It ended with her gripping my hand and looking at me in desperation. It's overwhelming, this frustration.

FEBRUARY 6: Today she watched Hillary Clinton declare her candidacy for U.S. senator from New York. Lois had been dozing, but when Hillary came on, I tell you she listened. I never saw her eyes more alert. She loves politics. She loves news. I remember how surprised, and delighted, I had been when we married and I discovered her interest. She had a bulky collection of cartoons. The political cartoons dated from FDR's first term, but she also had dozens of cartoons dealing with the war in Europe.

In late 1945, or early 1946, I had tried to parlay the best of these "war cartoons" into a book entitled *A Cartoon History of World War II*.

I almost pulled it off. I had become a friend of Prosper Bruanelli, ace writer for Lowell Thomas (one of the country's foremost newscasters at that time), and Prosper was a close friend of Dick Simon, with whom Max Schuster founded Simon and Schuster. Prosper had edited crossword puzzles for the old *New York World*. It was with his help that these two recent graduates of Columbia University published their first book, a collection of crossword puzzles.

Prosper fixed it so that I got in to see Schuster, who examined with considerable interest my two sample chapters dealing with the Battle of Britain and the Allied invasion of France. Schuster called in Simon to have a look, and, although they made no commitment, I left the conference encouraged. But nothing came of it. They lost interest after learning that a similar book featuring the work of the noted British cartoonist David Lowe was about to be published.

FEBRUARY 12: She asked me something. I have no idea
what because it was just noise, but I faked it. I said,
"Yes," whereupon she burst out laughing.
"Caught me?" I asked.
She nodded and laughed harder, and *I* started
laughing. I'd love to know what it was. Must have been
a beaut.

FEBRUARY 16: Today I found a pair of barber's scissors I
hadn't seen for years, and remembered there was a
time in the 1980s when Lois cut my hair. She
volunteered to do it and I went along, not because of
money saved but because she would be fooling with
my hair—what was left—and I would be enjoying the
sensuality of it, my beloved touching me. She did this
for at least two years, a towel secured by a safety pin

about my shoulders, as she delicately snipped, and I considered how wonderful it was to have someone like her, loving, taking care of me.

The discovery of the barber's scissors reminds me of the day, not Christmas or a birthday, she came back from shopping with a pair of scissors for me—scissors with ten-inch blades, the kind editors use for cutting whole pages out of newspapers. She knew, of course, my propensity for clipping, and she presented me with this outsized pair of scissors so happily I feigned delight, for, in truth, I had little use for it. The stories I clip from newspapers and magazines are so much shorter than this pair was designed for. I said nothing of that. What I feel guilty about now is that I didn't sometimes use the scissors (when she could see me using them) to please her. It would have been such a little thing to do.

FEBRUARY 17: I'm sneaking her an occasional cup of coffee—when we're alone in the apartment. She enjoys coffee so, and what harm can it do?

FEBRUARY 18: I'm touched by how she lets me take charge. If I'm wheeling her through a narrow space I say, "Pull in your elbows," and she pulls them in. If she fails in performing and I say, "Try again," she will try again. If she's slumped in the wheelchair and I say, "Get yourself back up," she will try. She has placed herself in my hands. The trust is humbling.

On the walls of our apartment we have Chinese scrolls; a large hand-painted portrait of a mandarin; a print by Montague

Dawson, the famous seascape painter; and, of course, family photographs. But above all these, excepting family pictures, Lois enjoys a painting we bought years ago in Montreal. It shows a group of caribou, three going one way, and the fourth heading determinedly the other way. The independent fellow delights Lois and she names the picture a favorite. I report this because, as they say, "That's just like her to do that."

FEBRUARY 22: Alone with Lois in the elevator, I told her I loved her, and she said, clearly, with good pauses between each word, "I love you, too." I had thought I would never hear those words again.

FEBRUARY 24: She took forever going to sleep last night. "Look," I said, "you're supposed to be sleeping, not just lying there admiring your husband." She broke into that wonderful, sonorous laugh that came only with her illness. Asleep, she was still smiling.

MARCH 1: She still wants to help, to share as much as she can. I was refastening my wristwatch and she reached to help. I cry inside.

MARCH 2: This afternoon we took another nap together. With her so weak and me no Goliath, it was a struggle to get her on the bed. She went to sleep almost at once. I lay awake looking at her. Again, her face was the picture of utter contentment. I couldn't stop looking.

I thought of trying this one more time—one more time, I kept telling myself—but I doubted I could pull it off. I had hurt my back rather badly this time, and she had lost so much strength I was afraid that I might let her fall getting her from the wheelchair to the bed. So this precious thing we did twice never happened again.

MARCH 5: I'm proud of Lois, the way she has kept her sense of humor despite what she knows. Today, though, it got her in trouble. We were in her ward watching the video of a tenor singing popular songs from the 1920s and 1930s. When the title "Give Me a Little Hug, Honey" appeared on the screen, I read it to Lois, whereupon she leaned over from her wheelchair to hug me.

"It's the *title*," I said.

That made her choke on the custard she was eating. She strangled until an aide applied the Heimlich maneuver.

MARCH 10: I told her about the meeting with Hana Lane, my editor at Wiley, and she looked up at me from her pillow and said, "I . . . am . . . proud . . . of you." How that went to my heart!

Mrs. Lane and I had met in New York to discuss the publication of my father's biography, a work in which Lois had always believed.

MARCH 14: Lois is weakening. As she lay in bed tonight, she had a look of great weariness. There are shadows under her eyes I don't remember ever seeing before.

2000

MARCH 20: Finished putting everything together for the taxman. For more than forty years Lois prepared our income tax returns without the help of an accountant. Being incompetent with numbers, I'm overwhelmed even with help.

"If you don't see me for a while," I said to her, "it will be because I'm in federal prison."

She laughed. She still laughs at my dumb jokes.

MARCH 28: Thank you, God, for my beloved Lois.

MARCH 29: Lois fell today. She was sitting in a chair in the Alzheimer's ward and leaned too far to take hold of something. No bone broken, but she has a cut above her right eye. Aide James praised her "stoicism."

MARCH 30: Lois said, "I love you." It has been such a long time since she said that, I had given up.

APRIL 1: April Fool's Day, so I knelt before her and said amorously, "There's something I haven't done for a long time." She leaned toward me, lips pursed. "Yes," I said, "I haven't had a haircut for months." You can bet we kissed even so.

APRIL 2: Lois and I committed a naughty little cocktail party in the apartment. She enjoyed a glass of prohibited sherry, and I fixed a dandy of a martini. We had a really good time.

APRIL 8: Today I gave up Lois's garden box with its roses, peppermint, and daisies. We have both had boxes, but now another resident needs hers. Maybe ripping her nameplate off the box didn't hurt.

APRIL 9: I got a scare this Sunday. We were watching the Masters when Lois seemed to be no longer with me: instead of looking at the television, she was looking at her feet. When I stooped and looked up into her face, her eyes had no expression. She did not respond when I spoke. I checked quickly to see if she was breathing. She was, but for a few seconds I didn't know. When *60 Minutes* came on, so did she. At bedtime she was all right, but I feel now there is a snake in the garden.

APRIL 13: The episode has not recurred, but she is listless.

APRIL 15: Often when we are in the apartment I have to take Lois to the bathroom. She is no longer able to wipe herself. I am surprised how naturally I have taken to this, grateful I can do it, a feeling that is biblical, almost like washing her feet.

Morrie, the stricken professor in Mitch Albom's *Tuesdays with Morrie*, confides that what he dreads most as he weakens is the day when he can no longer wipe himself. Lois, submitting to my ministrations, showed no sign of embarrassment. I have wondered about our reactions, and decided she reacted this way because she was a common-sense person and because we had become so much a part of each other.

APRIL 18: My flower box has a new nameplate, "LOIS AND ED BLISS." As long as I'm around, that will stay.

APRIL 19: In the woods Lois's wheelchair struck a hole filled with fresh dirt, pitching her onto the ground. After checking for injuries, a fellow resident, Bob Boardman, and I got her back in the chair. I reported the accident to nurse Naz. She gave Lois a thorough going-over and, probably because of the soft dirt, found no injury. Lois stoops so far forward in the chair now; I'm going to have to be more careful.

APRIL 23 (Easter): Anne and Tom came loaded with good Chinese food, which the four of us ate in the apartment. While we were eating, two Chinese American friends Rita and H. T. Huang dropped by with two magnificent Easter lilies, about the largest I've ever seen. They join a beautiful lily Anne brought last week.

APRIL 25: So much that is wonderful happens that I can't describe—like Lois's expression when I kiss her. She smiles like a schoolgirl, a mix of mischievousness and delight.

APRIL 27: Every day I throw away something she used. Today it was a small aluminum cup for mixing ingredients such as flour and water. You shook it with the lid on and, because of its shape, the ingredients blended. She bought it when we set up housekeeping. It was so clever—neat, she said—and she loved it. I lost the lid and now I have let the cup go. You wouldn't think a thing like that could hurt.

MAY 1: Took a heavy punch today. Came up from lunch to find a message on my machine from Courtney, the social worker. She had called to tell me they are going to be reviewing Lois's plan of care on May 11. She said it came to the team's attention over the past couple days that there has been a significant change in Lois's condition, prompting them to do "a certain amount of paperwork and planning for care." Her message said, "I hope you can attend if at all possible because we will be talking about her level of care and her placement at that time. If you could give me a call back at your convenience, I would appreciate it. Thank you."

Translation: "We're going to be removing your wife from the Alzheimer's unit to the less attractive infirmary on the second floor." A real blow. No one had told me that Lois's assignment to the unit was temporary.

LATER MAY 1: Courtney called again. Date for team meeting reset for May 18.

MAY 3: In our goodnight prayer, which only I say now, I thanked God for the gift of love. I ended, "I'm so grateful," and in that dear, cracked voice of hers she said, "Me, too." They mean everything, those two words. The only words I have heard her say for days.

MAY 4: I took Lois into the garden. I wanted to show her that our Queen Elizabeth roses have bloomed, but she didn't raise her head to see them.

I said, "Honey, raise your head. They're pretty."

I thought she could raise her head if she really tried. Then I wondered: "Can you raise your head?" I asked.

Softly, as though sharing a confidence, she said, "No."

It was one of the last comprehensible words I ever heard her say.

MAY 5: Sometimes I lie down beside her. I can do this when she goes to bed on her right side and leaves enough room. If she is in the middle of the bed, I have to wait for another night. But usually I have room and, lying close, can put my right arm about her shoulders and left arm about her waist. Her waist shocked me the first time because it seems all bone.

It's strange how little I remember of the forty-two years we slept in the same bed. I recall love-making, turning my back to her when I had a cough, the welcome warmth of her body on cold nights. But these recollections are strangely rare. According to my arithmetic, we must have said our prayers together more than 18,000 nights, but I recall specifically, in detail, only one time: we had quarreled and agreed that praying together made it impossible to remain quarrelsome. It astonishes me. Why, out of so many events, do I remember so few? I want now to remember everything. I hunger to see her face, the look of her, when she was young. I see the young woman in photographs, but can't see her clearly in my mind.

MAY 6: I have invaded her space. There's room in her closets and mine are overflowing, so I have hung my winter things in one of hers. Seeing all the dresses she will never wear again, I cried out, *"I can't do it!"* But I did.

MAY 8: There's an audio tape we often play at bedtime, a montage of Tchaikovsky numbers taken from *The Sleeping Beauty* and *Swan Lake.* Orchestra and lovely piano; right for going to sleep.

MAY 10: Not much Lois can do now. They're feeding her, but she still understands everything; and I can't remember when she cried last.

MAY 11: We had a fine time in the woods, the breeze sweet on our faces.

MAY 12: Last night I told her I was lonesome, and immediately she raised her arms to me. That is what she has been like all these years. God has been awfully good to me.

MAY 13: I have to report this. We had a bathroom accident today that was a doozy. We were in the apartment and Lois, afflicted with diarrhea, had to go. I wheeled her in and, as usual, she took hold of the bar across from the john to help lift herself out of the wheelchair. I pulled down her slacks and, holding her, told her to let go of the bar. She had to let go because her arms are too short for her to hold onto the bar *and* sit.

I saw the first feces trickle on the floor. "Let go," I said. *"Let go!"* Because her responses are so slow now, she still grasped the bar, and there was a great dismaying outpouring.

"Holy shit!" I cried, and Lois burst out laughing.

"Not funny," I said.

But it was. This must be one of our worst experiences, and most amusing—thanks to Lois's sense of humor.

MAY 14: Mother's Day. Tom is with his mother in Dallas, but Anne came over with Andrew. She brought food so we could eat in the apartment. Took pictures. A good, precious time.

MAY 17: Pushing Lois this afternoon, I made a joke, but she didn't laugh—she always laughs. It frightened me. Had the Alzheimer's done something else to her? But when I went around in front of her and looked up into her face, I saw she was smiling. How good to see that smile! She hadn't been stricken further; she just hadn't laughed out loud.

MAY 18: Anne and I met with Bobbie Beharrie, the capable head nurse of the Alzheimer's unit, and other caretakers to discuss Lois's transfer to the infirmary. The move will be tomorrow at 9:30 A.M., and Lois will be back in the same room, 208. I made a speech: I told them that, for God's sake, in the future they should tell family members that assignment to the marvelous, state-of-the-art Alzheimer's unit is temporary; that

when patients become helpless, they will be transferred.
I said I had taken great comfort in the thought that
Lois would be there until the end. I had been relieved
to think she wouldn't have to move yet again, and that
she would be comfortable in the room we had chosen
for her. They expressed regret for what had happened—
Lois was among the first patients taken into the unit,
before things had been worked out. Criteria for care
there have been established now. Family members are
being informed.

MAY 19: Turns out Lois wasn't moved until noon. Before
that I took down pictures, greeting cards, etc. Found
her crying bitterly when I returned from lunch. I fixed
that by bringing her up to the apartment where we had
a quiet time together—she has never cried in the
apartment. I telephoned my friend Bill Hamilton,
chairman of the Resident Services Committee, which I
had joined, to tell him I would be unable to attend the
committee meeting scheduled for 2:30. As usual, I
stayed with Lois at bedtime. She seems at peace now.

MAY 20: Lois's roommate is Mary Ostryzcki, who,
thankfully, doesn't turn up the volume on her television.
She is friendly and has told me at least four times—I'm
not exaggerating—that she was married in London at
the age of fifteen. Anne gave up her precious Saturday
to come over and help her mom get settled.

MAY 21: Room 208 looks out over a low roof. From Lois's
pillow the view is of a brick wall, but when wheeled to

the window, which faces east, she sees the South Woods and the sky. I have hung up family pictures and the colorful Bar Harbor poster she enjoyed in her old room. Mary Ostryzcki spends most of the day in a stuffed chair facing the window. Lois doesn't seem to mind the change. "Are you all right?" I ask, and every time, softly, like a breath, she says, "Yes."

MAY 23: I have sent a note to Goodwin House administrators expressing gratitude for the excellent care Lois received in the Alzheimer's unit. I praised individual nurses and nurse's aides by name. I found them both competent and caring. I can't say the same for the aides where Lois is now. In the Alzheimer's ward, a nurse's aide brushed Lois's hair when she got up from a nap. Not here, not so far. Last night an aide pulled off Lois's shoes without untying the laces. Tonight I found she had been put to bed wearing her necklace and earrings. No smile from the aide who tends her most. No hug or hands on Lois's shoulders to show caring.

Later I encountered aides who did show caring. I believe Goodwin House recruited the best aides it could. Because of the growing number of rest homes and life-care centers, demand for aides has exceeded supply. You hire the most capable you can. The RNs who saw Lois are first rate. I was particularly impressed by Tony Abamgie, who is from Nigeria, and Alberta Akrong.

MAY 24: It is with heavy heart that I visit Lois now. She sits crumpled in her wheelchair, no longer able to speak, scarcely able to move. When I sit with her I no longer see her face. The head so bent down.

MAY 25: Again I found Lois on the far side of the bed, so I could lie beside her. She went to sleep, and I almost did, to strains of *Swan Lake*.

MAY 27: They still don't untie her shoes; a small thing, I suppose, but I spoke to Tony.

MAY 28: Tonight her shoelaces were untied.

MAY 29: We prayed together, her lips barely moving, the small prayer we made up that ends, "and we thank you for this day." It is a prayer that we often prayed through the years, but tonight when we came to thanking, it was too much. Her eyes were shut, so she didn't see me crying.

JUNE 1: I said to her, "Isn't it *something* to have a love affair that lasts sixty years?" She seemed, from her expression, to take pleasure in the thought.

JUNE 2: Tonight, waiting for Lois to be prepared for bed, I played solitaire with her watching, the wheelchair drawn close. When I shuffled the cards and handed them to her to cut, she reached over most naturally and cut them. It was a small act, but big to me. I could almost believe a miracle had been performed, that she was going to be healed.

JUNE 5: We still kiss at the kissin' places, but now,
with her head bowed, I have to kneel in front of
the wheelchair to kiss her. When I accuse her
of holding her head down this way just so I have to
get down on my knees to her, she's tickled. I
think I'm trying to get all the kisses I can while it's
still possible.

JUNE 6: Attending tonight's piano recital, Lois
applauded ever so softly, even more softly than before.
She applauded devotedly after every piece. Difficult
not to cry.

JUNE 8: Told Lois I had changed the dedication of
Father's biography so it would be dedicated to her.
She looked pleased, but didn't speak. It is rare she *can*
speak.

JUNE 10: Lois's left hand has turned on itself, so bent that
all I can think of is a claw. Wrong on someone so dear. I
haven't mentioned this to Dr. Heinen; I'm sure he's
noticed.

JUNE 12: Beautiful day. Bright sun, low humidity.
Everyone I met at the dry cleaner's, post office, and
supermarket extremely friendly. I drove with the
window down, the June air caressing my face. From
the car radio came Mozart's magnificent Concerto in C
Major. I felt sublimely alive. Then, remembering Lois,
felt guilty.

JUNE 15: Today we did something different. I wheeled Lois into the garage, and she watched me wash our car.

JUNE 16: Something else different. I am reading *Daisy Miller* to her. I read it as we sit in the woods. I'm not sure I should have chosen James's sad story.

JUNE 18: All of a sudden Lois has no appetite. She ate almost nothing tonight, and it was the Sunday supper she likes. All she went for was the buttermilk.

JUNE 19: It wasn't lack of appetite: she can hardly swallow. I mean, swallow at all. For weeks they have been giving her pureed food. What's curious is that until yesterday she seemed to have little trouble eating what I gave her. Had my stir-fried chicken been so irresistible? Or had part of it been she made an extra effort to please me, the cook?

JUNE 20: She went to sleep smiling. I had told her that her beloved Red Sox are in first place. She often smiles. She smiles delightfully when I say, "May I kiss you?" Bless her heart.

JUNE 21: First day of summer, a hot and humid day, but we went outdoors anyway. We sat on our bench, and I read her more *Daisy Miller* and a sweet note from her sister, Jo, who writes every week. She also hears regularly from her niece Annie Mary Luke, who lives in North Carolina, and Jean Garnett, our friend in

Newbury, Massachusetts. Lois loves receiving these
letters and, I believe, understands every word.

JULY 1: She loves to hear the Red Sox have won. Her
favorite player is Garciaparra, not only because he can
hit, but because she enjoys the sound of his name,
especially when I stretch it out, "Gar . . . ci . . . a . . .
parra."

JULY 2: I was beside her, our heads touching, and started
singing the 1930s hit "Dancing Cheek to Cheek," then
made it "Sitting Cheek to Cheek." And there it was—I
could count on it—Lois's laugh, scarcely audible.

JULY 5: Went into the woods. Lois watched as I watered a
clump of coral-bells. They have tiny pink blooms. Lois
loves them. I take them to her from our garden box
and hate how their blooms drop off and scatter all over
the floor.
    I pretended to turn the hose on Lois, directing the
stream ever closer. She showed no concern. She looked
at me calmly with a boys-will-be-boys expression,
knowing that there was no way I would douse her. I
told her I never teased a girl I didn't like. But this is no
time for teasing.

JULY 8: She's beyond saying goodnight now. Her arms are
becoming petrified; they move with great difficulty. For
the first time, residents show shock at the sight of her
when we get the mail. We may have to stop doing that.

JULY 9: Sunday supper in the apartment, and Lois ate a
fair helping. Nurses say that she recently has been
eating hardly anything, and with the weight she's
lost—almost forty pounds now—I believe it.

This was our last supper together in the apartment. The next
Sunday, July 16, was Lois's birthday, and Anne and Tom ate
with us in a small dining room reserved for patients and guests.
By the next Sunday, Lois would be bedridden. The Sunday after
that, she would be gone.

JULY 11: Today when we went into the woods I remembered to bring peanuts. Three squirrels—two gray, one
black—and my Lois had a time. We must do this again.

JULY 13: I don't think I can describe this, how wondrous it
was, or what it means to me. As usual, coming in from
the woods for Lois's supper, I had wheeled her to a
table. As usual, I had told her I would be back at
bedtime and left. Then the wonderful, unusual thing
happened. When I turned at the elevators and looked
back, Lois very slowly, with great difficulty, was raising
her arm. I saw her bring it to her chin, then to her
mouth, then toward me. From the far end of the
room—across all the tables, patients, and nurse's
aides—my sweetheart was blowing me a kiss. I thank
God I looked back. How awful if I hadn't.

JULY 14: Lois fell from her wheelchair. Just toppled,
possibly reaching for something. Thankful—very
thankful—for no injury.

JULY 16: Lois's eighty-ninth birthday. We had a little
party. Anne brought a cake, and Tom brought balloons
of all colors, which gave the room a festive air. Anne
opened and read numerous greetings. Lois took it all
in, but ate pitiably little. Every moment precious.

JULY 17: Things moved quickly this sad day. Again, Lois
was unable to eat any of her breakfast, even though it
was pureed. A nurse suggested that she might have to
be fed intravenously. The suggestion, despite what I
know, comes as a shock. This afternoon when Anne
came to wash Lois's hair, we had a long talk and arrived
at the painful decision to place Lois in hospice care. So
that's how it will be now. Hard to believe that finally,
what we knew would come, has come.

Anne, rescuing me from the task, telephoned Dr.
Heinen's office but could not reach him. When he
called back, Anne had left. He advised me that if Lois
took food directly into her stomach, through a tube,
she would regain energy and possibly live for months. I
said, in words sentencing to death my dearest person,
that neither Anne nor I would want that for ourselves
and were sure Lois wouldn't either. She has signed
papers saying that, if in a terminal condition, she
wanted "no prolongation of life by unnatural means."
Dr. Heinen said he would instruct staff to take only
those measures deemed necessary for Lois's comfort.

When I went to see Lois at four o'clock I was
happy—so happy I said, "Thank you, God"—for I
found her in her wheelchair fully dressed. It meant we
could go as usual to get the mail—there were *seven*

personal letters, a record—and go to our place in the woods. The air had been cleared by morning rain; the sun seemed, more than ever, to give Lois's hair the radiance of silver.

We were there together for only a short time before I started crying. I put my head in her lap and just let go. I felt her hand on my head, touching softly the top of my bald head, repeatedly touching. Comforting. And I had just shortened her life.

JULY 18: This morning Anne and I met with the managers of Goodwin House's hospice program, Joyce Bramson and Cindy Nothom. I was impressed by them and sorry to hear that Bramson is leaving for another position. There will be, they said, papers for me to sign. After this meeting, which ended at ten-thirty, I went down to Lois and found her in bed. No more wheelchair, no more getting the mail together, no more excursions into the woods. It has happened all of a sudden and forever.

JULY 19: The hospice nurses have taken over. When I went down to see Lois this morning, two of them were bathing her. When they left, we spent a long time holding hands. Lois, dear heart, seems unable to utter a single word. I'm broken.

JULY 21: Lois stayed in bed all day, too weak for even the wheelchair. Dr. Heinen examined her. I watched the tall doctor stoop over her, taking her pulse, listening to her heart. Then he came over to me and said, very quietly,

"She's ready to go." Because of the way the doctor spoke, and perhaps, too, because death had been so long coming, his words produced a sense of acceptance.

Kate Jenkins, a seminary student, came and read Psalms to Lois in a most beautiful way. I stood in the doorway listening. It was unthinkable to break in.

The scene of Kate Jenkins sitting there reading Lois's beloved Psalms, interrupting herself every little while to stroke Lois's hair, lives with me. Lois lay on her side facing the seminary student, listening with a thirst. I watched from the doorway for a long time. It was too precious a picture to lose readily.

After dinner and a visit with Lois, I walked out into the woods and, sitting on our bench, thought how quickly it had happened. Nothing was changed in the woods—the bench, the squirrels, the crows, the birdbath someone must have just filled. In the twilit sky the treetops formed the same circle. Three days earlier I had no idea we were sitting together there for the last time. (Shouldn't we know when we are doing things like that?) When I returned to the infirmary at seven-thirty Lois was asleep. On her bedside table was a book about the discovery of climber George Mallory's body on Mt. Everest. I had been reading it to her and now, beside her bed, I read to myself. I stayed until a little after ten. She was still sleeping peacefully when I left.

JULY 22: Saw Lois shortly after nine this morning. She was sleeping with her eyes half open. When I returned an hour later Anne and Tom were with her, together with Kate Jenkins and Cindy Northom from Hospice. Cindy said Lois was "handling it well." In late morning I found Kate again at Lois's bedside reading the Psalms, again stopping every so often to look at Lois and, very softly, stroke her hair. I went to lunch and then, after finding Lois sleeping, took a nap. In late afternoon I read to Lois and watered our garden box. Tonight, precious telephone calls from Alison in Connecticut and Andrew in Tennessee. They wanted to know how "Lady" is.

JULY 23: An aide was working over Lois. By habit I went to her, but was unprepared for what I saw. She lay naked, the picture of a body from Buchenwald, and I quickly withdrew. That was at 10:15 A.M. As I waited in the small library across from Lois's room, I heard the aide call for a nurse. That scared me, but it was only the aide needing help to turn Lois over.

JULY 24: Anne, bless her heart, was here most of the day. She could do that because she and Tom have abandoned their plan to spend the week vacationing. Bob Edwards dropped by on his way home from NPR, and I'm pretty sure Lois knew it was Bob and appreciated his coming. Dear James Barber, the aide who got to know Lois well in the Alzheimer's ward, came to tell Lois, "God bless you." Anne startled me by saying, "I've said goodbye to Mom." She believes that will help Lois "let go." Anne is a hospice nurse so knows more than I do, but I can't do that. Not yet.

At five o'clock Kate was back. All day Lois had shown no interest in anything going on around her, but now she listened to Kate with interest. I'm grateful to Kate, who, with her gentleness and understanding, will be a splendid priest, I know.

I was sitting with Lois after Kate left when I saw her
body stiffen. It stiffened from head to foot, and her dear
face took on the expression of someone trying to lift a
great load. Her features were all distorted, contorted, and
then, as I leaned toward her anxiously, she let out without
doubt the ugliest human sound I have ever heard—
a three-syllable sound wrung from her whole body, a
last supreme effort to speak. We both burst into tears.

I remember grabbing her and crying, "I know, honey. I know.
I know." But the pain. She had demanded of herself a voice,
three words, which I do believe were "I love you," and failed.
I did not hear words, only awful sounds, and what hurts is that
she heard them. By the measure of her sobs, her heart was
breaking. I treasure the gift she wanted to give. Knowing her,
I would not be surprised if she had planned the effort, calcu-
lated the risk, and daringly decided to try.

JULY 25: I will tell people she died last night at ten
    minutes to ten. That is when I looked at my watch and
    realized she was gone. Anne and Tom were with me.
    They stood on one side of the bed and I on the other. A
    small teddy bear wearing a blue sweater lay on Lois's
    breast. We knew it would not be long. As early as
    seven-thirty that evening, before Anne and Tom came,
    her breath had been coming in gasps. I held her hand
    and prayed aloud the "Now I Lay Me" we prayed as
    children. I rearranged her covers (she had too much
    cover) and sang "In the Garden," her favorite bedtime
    song, and kissed her and told her I loved her. In fixing
    the bedcovers I discovered that her left hand, which had

seemed permanently clenched, was now relaxed. At
seven-forty a terrorizing rattle came from her throat.
"Oh, God, no!" I cried, "Not *that!*"

This is when Anne and Tom came, and Anne
immediately ordered a drug "to ease the breathing."
Exhausted, I went to the apartment to lie down, but
within minutes Anne telephoned, "Mom is slipping
away," and I ran down the stairs to her. The three of us
stood by Lois's bed, caressing her and crying as slowly
she left us. Even then, after she was gone, I held her
hand. I could not let go. I got out of the room when
they came to take her. I wanted none of that.

Her eyes turned a deeper blue when she died. They were clear
as a girl's and astonished me with their expression. It was as
though, in the last functioning of her mind, she had been fascinated by the experience, as though something interesting and
not at all scary was happening. I was astonished. I said to Anne,
"Did you see what I saw?" and she said, "Yes, Dad, I did."

JULY 27: The sky began crying when Lois died and now,
after three days of mourning, the sun has come out in
its glory. It lights the tops of the trees in our woods
with a light I have never seen before. It has turned the
wet tops of trees to silver—how can it do that?—
against a gray sky, a lovely gray, making a celebration.

———⸙———

That was my last entry. The next day a letter from Cronkite
brought me close to crying. I had sent him a picture of Lois

taken on Mother's Day, and his first words were: "I was much encouraged to see the photo of Lois. She looks so much better than I had expected." He said he was sorry not to visit. "On Monday, I undergo surgery to repair a torn tendon in my leg." The letter ended, "Give Lois my love."

We held the memorial service in Goodwin House chapel, and as they used to say in obituaries, it was "largely attended." Anne spoke of how her mother's life "reflected her innermost values of love, generosity, courage, loyalty to family, and service to others. I am honored," she said, "that this lovely lady told me that I was a good daughter. I have her to thank for the qualities that made it possible." I read the brave letter Lois wrote to her sister upon being diagnosed as having Alzheimer's disease, and a note from the seminary student Kate Jenkins who wrote of "the light of Christ" in Lois's eyes as she lay dying. And I read the poem I had written on her last birthday:

Say it in the simplest way, they say.
Do not adorn.
So now I simply say
God bless this day
That you were born.

I have in you
All glory,
All recompense,
And faith, Dear Heart,
That you and I
In deepest sense
Shall never part.

I said it's not true, of course, but I always felt she was the most wonderful woman in the world.

Together we read the Twenty-third Psalm and sang Lois's favorite hymn, "In the Garden," which I had dared sing to her so many times.

Lois would have been pleased that former students came—she loved them as I did—and delighted that her niece Annie Mary and her husband, Ed Luke, were there, having driven up from Wagram out of love for her. The small Carolina town of her childhood was represented, after all.

On September 16, in glorious sunlight, Lois's ashes were interred in Newburyport next to the ashes of the younger daughter she had lost. Just as I had always taken a single, long-stemmed rose to her whenever she was hospitalized, I placed a long-stemmed red rose on her grave.

In this way, it ended.

Epilogue

The next spring I returned to Newburyport. At the cemetery I had trouble finding precisely where in our lot they had interred Lois's ashes. Then, finding it, I laid across the sod another long-stemmed rose, bright red. After a week visiting good friends in this city where we had spent our happiest years, I drove again to the cemetery as I was leaving. I stood looking at the rose that was now wilted, at the graves of my parents and the daughter we had lost, at the future grave for me, and I could just imagine Lois being touched, and a little amused, that I had felt compelled to come back to her once more before leaving town. I heard myself saying out loud, "But, honey, you *knew* I would." Then, crying bitterly, I said goodbye.

I was used to crying. I had discovered that *heartache* is no figure of speech. The heart does ache; can ache so it hurts. All around me were reminders producing this hurt: the Chinese rug she chose; her writing desk; the photograph of her taken in Paris on our tenth wedding anniversary; the coffee table she gave me that I had varnished black, hoping it would look like lacquer; the little bronze pony she prized. The month after Lois died I was cleaning out a drawer and discovered a plastic envelope full of her handkerchiefs and, taped onto it, this note:

Judging by the handwriting, uncorrupted by Alzheimer's disease, the note must have been written before 1996. Because this was Lois looking after me again, and telling me she loved me, I wept.

In the residents' dining room I could see where we had eaten breakfast together each morning for eight years. I visualized her after eating, hurrying off to exercise class while I stayed for another cup of coffee. She never could get me to go with her. I wish I had. I wish I could go back and do this over.

The reminders seemed unbearable. One day I stood in our bedroom looking at her bed, and screamed. I was in pain. C. S. Lewis said losing his wife was like having a leg cut off again and again. I have seen obituaries saying, "He never recovered after his wife's death."

Even though they were at times unbearable, I must say the reminders around me also gave comfort. I would have fought to keep the little pony and other tokens; they are a part of Lois I still have.

Everyone was kind. When I went down to breakfast the first morning, two waitresses took me in their arms. Fellow residents said, "You have such memories," though the memories seemed then only to underscore the loss. Others, comforting me, said we would be together in heaven. Lois and I knew there is no hell except what we make for ourselves, and knew so little of heaven, we trusted God for it. We believed if heaven existed, it had to be a grand celebration of the spirit. We did not rule it out.

We had no belief in resurrection of the body, the marvelous apparatus for life on earth. Our image of God appeared in self-less love and nature's glories, from the firefly's wee light to the grandeur of the mountains. We liked best God's Native American name, Great Spirit, for God is a spirit so illustrious in wisdom and love as to be incomprehensible, yet recognizable in wonderful works; remote as the most distant star, yet intimate as breathing. Lois left everything up to the Great Spirit who had been good to us.

Because of this trusting, agnostic attitude, I did not have the comfort enjoyed by others who are confident of joyful reunion after death. But not a day passed I did not thank God for Lois and what we had.

Part of me could not comprehend Lois had died. When I passed the door to the Alzheimer's unit, I had the feeling that if I went in, she would be there; that if I went to our bench and just waited, she would come. Sometimes in the apartment, seeing the vacant space where she had sat in her wheelchair, I felt I could still bring her up from the second floor if only I had faith and went down there believing.

It's odd how I was affected by the deaths of famous people who died that same year: celebrities such as musical comedy stars Gwen Verdon and Julie London; the fine actors Walter Matthau and Alec Guiness, whom Lois enjoyed so much; dancer Gene Kelley; and the much-loved cartoonist Charles Schulz. I took no comfort in the deaths of these people; it's just the feeling that Lois hadn't gone alone.

I had thoughts I'd never had before. I wondered at the death of a wife much loved and how different it is from the death of a much-loved parent or child. In a good marriage the death of a husband or wife is the loss of a comrade with whom life has been shared intellectually, emotionally, sexually, spiritually. Totally.

I had bad thoughts. I caught myself thinking, "Why is that woman alive and not Lois? She's a vegetable." Or, I sometimes thought the same thing about some woman not a vegetable, but a terrible woman no one liked. I was ashamed of these thoughts. I didn't hold onto them.

Often now when I see couples rejoicing in their love, I think not of their joy but of the heartache waiting to happen, knowing from experience that the greater the love, the greater the pain on parting. I'm not sure this is a good thought either.

Lois was gone six months, half a year, and still at four in the afternoon I had the impulse to go to the second floor to see her. I still went for the mail a little after four, as we had done so many times, and I couldn't see the clock's hands at five o'clock without thinking how, sitting with her in the woods or in the apartment, this was the time I had said, "We have to go now, honey," because that was when the aides began serving supper. Eight o'clock was another time my life was set to: I missed the bedtime visits most.

I still used pharmaceuticals she had bought, and I dreaded the day I would take the last aspirin or use the last Band-Aid or Stim-U-Dent. The Stim-U-Dents worried me most, I suppose, because Lois had introduced me to them. When I got down to the last one, what would I do? Could I bring myself to use it? My solution—and this is ridiculous, I know—was to use none I had left, but buy a new supply. I bought one hundred—four packs— and put them on top of Lois's last pack, which I shall never use.

In her medicine cabinet, in neat rows, still stand her most intimate possessions, from bobby pins to Cardizem, to the small bottle of Chanel No. 5 perfume, mostly full although I gave it to her four years ago. And I find, unexpectedly, new reminders: an almost-empty bottle of nail polish; the bottom of her winter pajamas that somehow got into my bottom bureau drawer; an old lipstick, just the color she liked, the color she found hard to find. I discovered a used Kleenex in one of my overcoat pockets. I hadn't used it; she had—it bore the rosy imprint of her mouth. They catch me unaware, these other reminders that C. S. Lewis, after his wife's death, called "the tiny, heartbreaking commonplace."

I don't know precisely the turning point, but one day about a year after Lois died I realized I wasn't crying anymore. Instead of looking at her large studio portrait and sometimes breaking down, I was saying things like "Your Queen Elizabeth bush is blooming its head off," and, "Honey, the damnedest thing happened today." The last time Lois and I went to get the mail, I wheeled her around to where she could see the flowerbed in front of Goodwin House. I saw the flowerbed every day after she died. Every day it saddened me. Now it doesn't. I think of it as a good thing we shared.

Once in a while the pain returns, caused by something as ordinary as a box of Kleenex. We kept one in our car between us on the front seat, the mileage of many trips scribbled over the top of it. Returning from Anne's one day, I pulled out the last tissue, blew my nose, and when I got home, threw away the box—the ordinary, dutiful, now useless companion of our journeys. I hadn't cried for weeks, but I did over that lousy box. Another time, looking for the flashlight we kept in the glove compartment, my heart seemed to stop when, for the first time in a very long while, I saw the little round tin of assorted candies she used on long trips when her mouth was dry. I threw it away, too. They hurt, these small partings with the past.

I still haven't stopped doing things that are crazy, either—I just do them less often. Walking through the lobby, I saw an empty wheelchair. When no one was looking, I went over and took hold of its handles. The feel of them, so intimately associated with Lois, brought her close. Another time, again in the lobby, I had the thought that if I just stepped out in the sunshine, I could see the spun silver of her hair; I'd see it if I went outside.

I see her everywhere—so many reminders—happily now more often than sadly. An old song comes to mind:

> *I see your face in every flower,*
> *Your eyes in stars above.*
> *It's just the thought of you,*
> *The very thought of you,*
> *My love.*

C. S. Lewis spoke of falling in love with the memory of his wife. I think I've done that.

On the bench I think of her less sadly. Down by my feet, on the path, I see where her wheelchair rested, where the wheels were. The path has not changed. Nothing around me has changed. Here we fed the squirrels, watched the sparrows bathe, wondered at the coronet the tops of oak trees made high above us. When I was crying, head in her lap, it was here she comforted me. And it is here I still find comfort; so I keep coming.

When I see her favorite chair I still see her in it, but less often. When I do things she did, such as shopping, I less often think of her. I have caught myself looking at a full moon without thinking of her at all, though not often. Still, she's with me. Yesterday, starting up the path to the woods, I looked up at the blue sky spread out above me and shouted, "Hello, sweetheart!" I had no thought of doing that. It just came because of the majesty of what I saw; because the wonder brought her close.

I play pretend. When a special sunrise takes me by surprise, I call her to come and see. When I can't find my keys, I'm apt as not to ask her help. And last night when her Red Sox won with a home run in the ninth, I said, "How about that, honey?" I make believe and it helps.

But oh, I miss her! I won't pretend I don't. I miss her companionship and her pulling down the back of my crew neck sweater when I put it on. I miss her kisses and her scratching the itch I can't reach. I miss her embrace and her bringing me coffee as I work, her sewing buttons on and finding, magically, whatever I can't find. I think of how, each month or two, she took tweezers and plucked the one hair that keeps growing on the tip of my nose. I think of how she believed in me. I miss her clear, gray-blue eyes, her soft voice, her silver hair. I miss grievously her wise counsel. I miss her loving kindness.

I do not miss her love. It's all around me.

There are still things I cannot do. I cannot strip her bed. I do wash the counterpane and put on a fresh pillowcase every few weeks. But the sheets she had that last night of our life together, I leave as they were. Sometimes, not often, I touch them. I have none of her clothes—they have gone, sensibly, to the Salvation Army—but I have these sheets that were close to her, that her body warmed, that are just as they were. Nor can I remove the little white duck by the stove that's labeled "Lois's kitchen." These are too much a part of her for me to lose.

Most of my wounds now are self-inflicted. I don't *have* to stop by the Alzheimer's ward (to see the cat, I say); or when I visit a patient on the second floor, go around and look into the room where Lois died. (Old Mrs. Ostrzycki is still there, sitting the same way in the same chair.) Nor do I *have* to keep going back into the woods to our bench, but I do. I find peace as well as heartache in our Garden of Eden.

I see her in small portraits. I see her knitting booties for our babies, sewing on buttons, washing diapers. I see her carting groceries, putting them away, delighting in her newfangled pressure cooker. I see her ironing my shirts, refusing to iron my shorts, and frying chicken more delicious than any other fried chicken. I see her zipping the lining into my winter jacket so I'd be warm. I think of how, before doctors found the right medication for my arthritis, she knelt to tie my shoes.

I see her preparing the income tax. She did it without an accountant for forty-eight years and got not one call from the IRS. Only in the last years before she was stricken did she engage an accountant, and then he wondered why.

I think of her engagement picture, the photograph that appeared two columns wide in the paper because I was, after all, a member of the staff. I had slept, at that time, in my small "Y" room with the desk lamp on so I could see this photograph in the night. I still see it. She was looking slightly to the side. It was a face of gentleness and strength, with fine cheekbones, a purposeful chin, and eyebrows plucked according to the fashion of the time. And to think she would marry me!

Now, sixty-two years later, I look at this other picture on the living room wall, a picture taken after twenty years of marriage. Looking at that dear face, I sense she wasn't merely in a studio getting her picture taken. From this picture, she looks straight at you, deep into you. My strong belief is that, looking into the camera that day, she surmised that it might be the last formal picture taken of her, so she strove to show, by her expression, the love she had for us, all her family. I think how wonderfully she succeeded. I keep a light on no longer, but I do not go to bed at night without first visiting this picture on the wall and telling the lady in it that I love her, too.

I had pleasures with her in her illness that I did not realize I was having. Preparing those Sunday-night suppers was a pleasure. Fun, really. Wheeling Lois to our bench each fair day was routine, done partly out of duty, but now I see it was a most pleasant time. The realization of this came a few days after Lois died when I found I was no longer watching the Weather Channel or turning hungrily, with suspense, to forecasts in the morning paper. Weather didn't matter anymore. Neither rain nor snow could spoil our trysts now; Lois had left.

There was satisfaction—more than that, a sense of fulfillment—in doing things for her after all the years that, lovingly, she had done things for me. Big things, such as supporting me in my endeavors, and little things, such as cleaning my hair brush and squeezing orange juice—although, whether squeezing orange juice daily for more than half a century is a small thing is questionable. It had become my turn, and the feeling was good.

I still walk by our kissin' places and the wall she kept running into when she couldn't steer her walker. In the apartment I see by my chair the space that was hers when she was in her wheelchair. But instead of wounding me, these familiar places and sights give me comfort now. I've developed a fondness for them.

Alzheimer's disease robs its victims. Lois was robbed of the ability to read, write, walk, speak. Mercifully with her variation of Alzheimer's, she was allowed the ability to recognize and reason. But what if she had been unable to recognize anyone or had not been able to understand me?

I find the answer in what a man told me not long after Lois died. The man, in his seventies, was a volunteer with the local

Alzheimer's association, and he told me his wife had died of Alzheimer's. When I asked how long she had suffered with the disease, he said it was twelve years from the time she was diagnosed to the time she died. "The last three years," he said, "she didn't recognize me." He paused. His face brightened. "But," he said, "*I* recognized her." Despite everything, he had not been robbed of the person he loved.

In Mitch Albom's *Tuesdays with Morrie,* the thing that set me thinking most, and still reverberates, is the old professor's statement: "Love always wins." Could this be true? I didn't see how it could be, but now I think of the man who rejoiced in the fact that, although his wife could not recognize him, he, by God, could recognize her. The pure joy in his face showed that love had won. And I feel—I *know*—that love won with us, or how could I be so grateful?

I was reading an editorial in the *New York Times,* and a sentence—six words—leapt at me: "In time, grief turns into thanks." The editorial, entitled "Thanksgiving 2001," was referring to what the nation suffered that unforgettable September 11, but the sentence seemed written for me. Grief turning into gratitude wasn't so remarkable after all.

"Love suffereth long and is kind . . . is not puffed up . . . endureth all things," and, yes, transforms all things. So, now when I look back on what happened, including all the sadness, I see a love story. There is still heartache at times: I miss Lois too much for there not to be. But I *had* so much. People speak of real time; we had real life, and what was most real were the last years. In those years, more than any other, we were one.

In the end, what was cruel was no match for love.

Finis

AFTERWORD

My father did not live to see this book published. At the age of ninety, Dad was inflicted with a chronic lung condition that flared up unexpectedly; he collapsed in November 2002 and died a week later, just before Thanksgiving. He did receive the joyful news of the book's acceptance, and he did go to New York to meet the publishers and sign the contract—less than three weeks before his death. He felt a sense of mission about the book: "This is a story that needs to be told; this book will help others." He was thrilled about publication and the good he felt this story would do others. Writing it also helped him, bringing him through a grief that was so profound I did not think he would survive it.

Dad saw Mom as just about as perfect as a person can be. Their admiration of each other lasted a lifetime. I, too, enjoyed a lifelong admiration of Mom. Her life and mothering reflected her innermost values of love, generosity, spirituality, courage, loyalty to family, and service to others. That was her greatest gift to us.

Mom's great delight was her grandchildren, and much thought, joy, and love went into her relationships with them. Her oldest granddaughter, Lisa, began calling her "Lady" when she started talking, and all the grandchildren followed this tradition. This name was no coincidence—Mom was truly a lady.

Mom's manner to others was gentle and sweet, but as a mother and grandmother, she was also fiercely loyal and supportive of her family. She made a warm, loving home for my sister, Lois, and me. She never made comparisons between her daughters—a quality I didn't fully appreciate until I was grown. As a mother, of course, she knew best—even as an adult I learned to ignore her advice at my peril.

Mom enriched our lives with her sense of humor and wonderful storytelling. My sister and I loved hearing stories of Mom's girlhood growing up in North Carolina in a large family: stories about the time all the kids were on the back of the horse, and one slipped off over the tail; about seeing her first airplane; about the influenza epidemic of 1919; and, most fun, about how, during her undergraduate days, she had skinny-dipped in the fountain on her college campus.

Being a lady didn't mean Mom was prudish—her sense of humor sometimes ran to the risqué and earthy, occasionally to the embarrassment of my dad and the enjoyment of her children. This wonderful sense of humor we all loved was apparent in Mom even in the face of her terrible illness, right up until the last few weeks of her life.

Education was one of Mom's lifelong priorities. She often helped me with spelling lists, and I credit her tutoring with my getting through the math section of the College Boards. She had also been dedicated to the blind students she taught in North Carolina before her marriage. Her thoughtfulness, love, and loyalty were reflected in the gratitude of these students: several years ago, Dad was on the Larry King radio show being interviewed by Jim Bohannon, when one of Mom's students from more than fifty years earlier called in to warmly express his appreciation for her work.

Mom was an avid reader and wrote beautifully. These qualities and skills helped her be Dad's—"best"— editor. She gave him editing advice both on small details and major decisions of judgment. She was as fascinated as Dad by the news business, and felt that being informed was a necessity.

Mom was a courageous person—courageous to marry a Yankee and move north, strong through the sudden loss of her father in an accident when she was a young woman, and again when confronted with the untimely death of my sister, Lois. She was brave also in facing the suffering during her last illness.

Dad was grief-stricken after Mom's death. The publication of his father's biography six months later helped him to focus and function, as did the writing of this book. The emotional pain affected him deeply, but he never lost his zest for life: for upholding and promoting rigorous standards for his profession, broadcast journalism (in 2002 he was honored with an award for Distinguished Service in Local Journalism from the Washington, D.C. chapter of the Society of Professional Journalists); for his deep commitment to his family and friends; for teaching (he met with journalism students the month before he died); for his sense of adventure (the book he wrote about his childhood in China was, with good reason, entitled *Tom Sawyer in China*); for hard work (he was writing yet another book at the time of his death); and for his deep spiritual strength—a sense of gratefulness and graciousness. He continued to engage enthusiastically with his many interests after Mom died, but he told me several times that he had had a wonderful life and, when it was time for him to go, he would be ready.

At the end, Dad was as brave as Mom, accepting the prognosis of his sudden illness and insisting on being allowed to go forward to what was next on his own terms. After collapsing in November 2002, Dad learned the grim prognosis from his physician one evening, and the next morning he requested Hospice care. He asked us to honor his earlier decision not to be kept alive by artificial means. He said he was ready: "I want to go home; I don't mean Goodwin House." I believe he was surprised that he is now reunited with his beloved Lois.

Anne Mascolino